NCCN Guidelines for Patients®

The essential guide for people facing cancer.

Based on care recommendations from leading cancer experts.

Explains high-quality cancer care provided at state-of-the-art cancer centers.

Reviewed and revised every year.

Did you know that top cancer centers across the United States work together to improve cancer care? This alliance of leading cancer centers is called the National Comprehensive Cancer Network® (NCCN®).

Because cancer care is always evolving, NCCN develops and frequently updates evidence-based cancer care recommendations used by health care providers worldwide. These recommendations are known as the NCCN Clinical Practice Guidelines in Oncology (NCCN Guidelines®).

The NCCN Guidelines for Patients plainly explain these expert recommendations, so you can talk with your care team about the best care for you.

These NCCN Guidelines for Patients are based on the NCCN Guidelines® for Prostate Cancer, Version 5.2026 — January 23, 2026.

View the NCCN Guidelines for Patients free online: NCCN.org/patientguidelines

Find an NCCN Cancer Center near you: NCCN.org/cancercenters

Learn how the NCCN Guidelines for Patients are developed: NCCN.org/patient-guidelines-process

Connect with us

@NCCNorg @NCCNVideo NCCN @NCCNorg

Supporters

NATIONAL COMPREHENSIVE CANCER NETWORK®
NCCN FOUNDATION
Guiding Treatment. Changing Lives.

NCCN Guidelines for Patients are supported by funding from the NCCN Foundation®

NCCN Foundation gratefully acknowledges the following corporate supporters for helping to make available these NCCN Guidelines for Patients: AstraZeneca; Janssen Biotech, Inc.; and Novartis Pharmaceuticals Corporation.

NCCN independently adapts, updates, and hosts the NCCN Guidelines for Patients. Our corporate supporters do not participate in the development of the NCCN Guidelines for Patients and are not responsible for the content and recommendations contained therein.

To make a gift, visit
NCCNFoundation.org/Donate

To learn more, visit online
NCCN.org/patientguidelines
or email
PatientGuidelines@NCCN.org

Contents

NCCN Foundation seeks to support the millions of patients and their families affected by a cancer diagnosis by funding and distributing NCCN Guidelines for Patients. NCCN Foundation is also committed to advancing cancer treatment by funding the nation's promising doctors at the center of innovation in cancer research. For more details and the full library of patient and caregiver resources, visit NCCN.org/patients.

National Comprehensive Cancer Network (NCCN) and NCCN Foundation
3025 Chemical Road, Suite 100, Plymouth Meeting, PA 19462 USA

1

About early-stage prostate cancer

Everyone with a prostate has a chance of getting prostate cancer. It's usually not fatal, particularly early-stage prostate cancer. This chapter gives an overview of this common cancer and the ways to effectively manage it.

What is prostate cancer?

Prostate cancer is a disease where cells in the prostate gland multiply and grow out of control.

The prostate gland is located just below the bladder in the pelvis, deep inside of the area of your body between your hip bones. The prostate is an important part of the male reproductive system. This system also includes the penis, seminal vesicles, and testicles.

Prostate cancer is one of the most common types of cancer.

Cancer is what happens when something goes wrong with the natural cell process, causing some cells to multiply and spread.

Cancer cells don't behave like normal cells. Cancer cells develop genetic changes (mutations) that allow them to make many more cancer cells. They crowd out and overwhelm normal cells. This can end up harming the body.

Cancer cells survive much longer than normal cells do. They can replace many normal cells and cause organs to stop working well. Cancer cells can also spread outside of the prostate to other areas of the body.

Prostate cancer is described as either early-stage cancer or advanced-stage cancer.

The prostate gland is an important part of the male reproductive system. It's located in the pelvis, just below the bladder.

In a young adult, the prostate is normally about the size of a ping-pong ball. It grows larger with age.

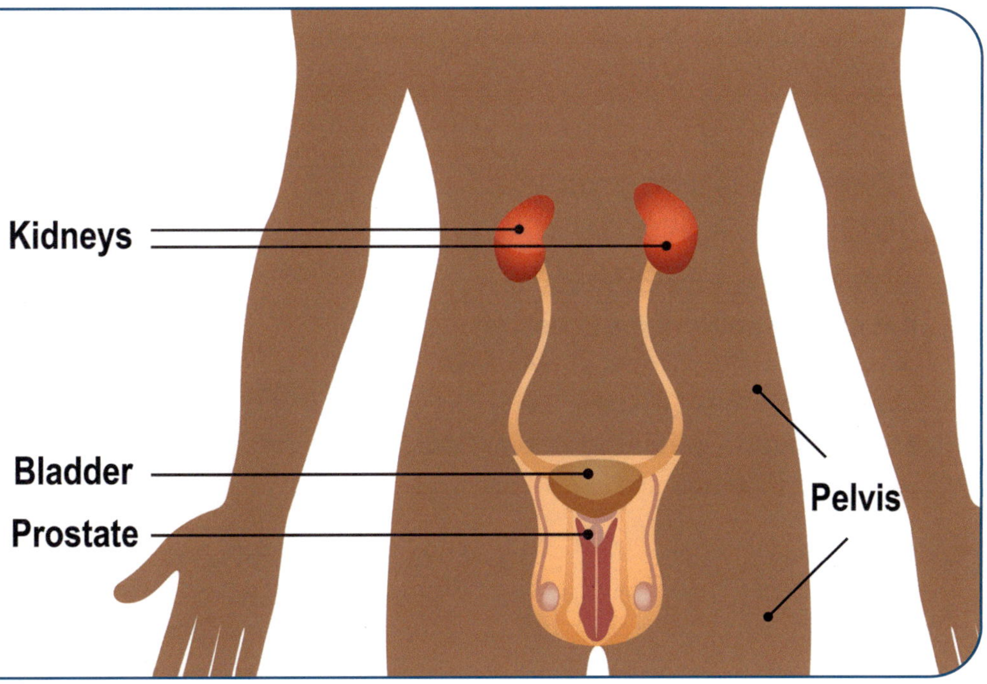

Early stage

Early-stage prostate cancer has not spread beyond the prostate gland. The cancer usually grows slowly and stays inside of the prostate. Cancer that is contained entirely within the prostate is also called localized prostate cancer.

Advanced stage

Advanced stage means that cancer cells have spread beyond the prostate to other areas in the body. This spreading is called metastasis or metastatic cancer. Metastatic prostate cancer may spread to lymph nodes, bones, liver, lungs, or other organs.

More information on advanced-stage prostate cancer is available at NCCN.org/patientguidelines and on the NCCN Patient Guides for Cancer app.

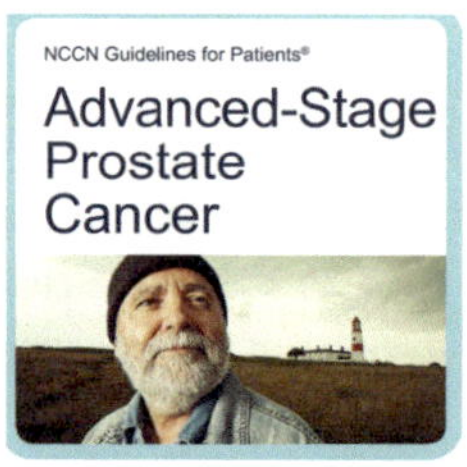

How is prostate cancer treated?

Recommended treatments for early-stage prostate cancer include active surveillance, surgery, radiation therapy, and hormone therapy.

Early-stage prostate cancer is highly treatable and often curable. The earlier that prostate cancer is diagnosed and treated, the more likely that a patient will live without cancer.

Scientists have learned a great deal about prostate cancer in recent years. As a result, today's improved detection methods and treatments work better than those in the past. There are also more treatment choices now than ever before.

However, many people with early-stage prostate cancer don't need to be treated immediately. What's more, most people with

What early-stage prostate cancer looks like

Early-stage prostate cancer has not spread beyond the prostate gland. It usually grows slowly and stays within the prostate. Early-stage prostate cancer is also called localized prostate cancer.

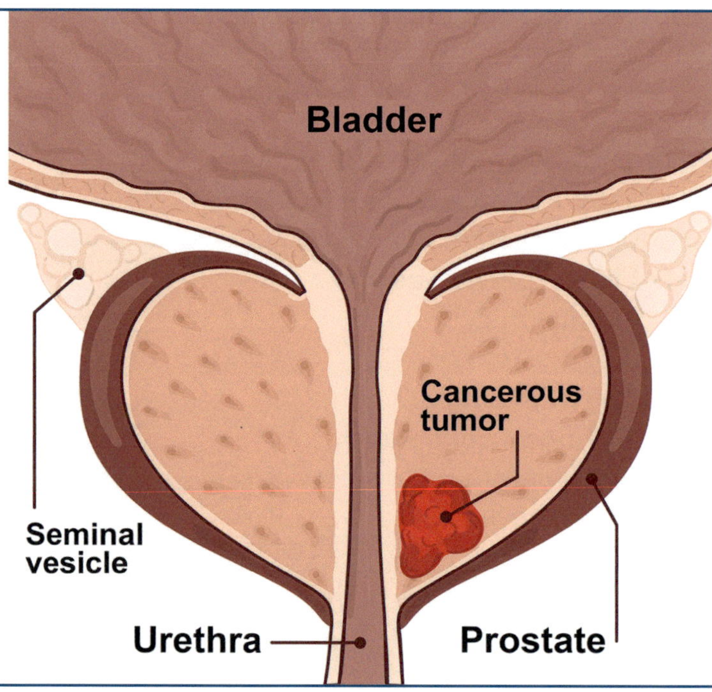

early-stage disease live without symptoms for many years and, in the end, usually die of something else.

Instead of immediate treatment, many people with early-stage prostate cancer can have their cancer managed initially with active surveillance.

During active surveillance, you'll have regular tests to keep an eye on your cancer. But you won't have treatment unless the cancer grows or changes in a way that requires some type of therapy.

The goal of active surveillance is to avoid the side effects of treatment, with the option for treatment in the future if you need it. Many people on active surveillance never need treatment.

How can I get the best care?

Advocate for yourself. You have an important role to play in your care. Many people feel more satisfied when they actively take part in planning their cancer care.

The NCCN Guidelines for Patients will help you play a larger role in your care. Discuss the recommendations in this guide with your care team. Ask questions about your options and share your goals and concerns.

Don't know what to ask? You're not alone. That's why we include suggested questions to ask at the end of chapters.

Keep reading to find the best care for you.

How this guide can help you

Making decisions about cancer care is stressful. There's a lot to learn, and you don't know what the future holds.

Use this guide to get the information and support you need.

Patients, doctors, and other health care professionals trust the NCCN Guidelines for Patients. This guide uses clear, everyday language to explain current cancer care recommendations made by respected experts in the field. Their recommendations are based on the latest research and practices at leading cancer centers.

Your health is unique to you, so your cancer care should be, too. As you read this guide, you'll learn which treatments are likely to provide the best results for you. And you'll be better prepared to talk with your care team.

"Now more than ever, those living with cancer are living better, longer lives thanks to the power of research and advancements in treatment."

2

Symptoms and risk factors for prostate cancer

Cancer researchers don't know exactly what causes prostate cells to become cancerous, but certain factors can increase your risk. People with prostate cancer usually have one or more of these risk factors.

Prostate cancer is the second most common cancer in American males and has one of the highest survival rates of any cancer when found early.

What are the symptoms of prostate cancer?

Prostate cancer often grows slowly and shows no symptoms for a long time. In fact, most people diagnosed with early prostate cancer have no noticeable symptoms.

Symptoms are more common in people with advanced prostate cancer.

If someone seems to have symptoms of early-stage prostate cancer, their symptoms are usually not from cancer but instead from an unrelated issue, like a condition called **enlarged prostate**.

Enlarged prostate (also called benign prostatic hyperplasia, or BPH) is much more common than prostate cancer. Enlarged prostate occurs in about half of males by 60 years of age. It becomes even more common as they grow older.

With BPH, the enlarged prostate can push against the bladder and compress the urethra. This slows the flow of urine and can cause a feeling that you haven't fully emptied your bladder.

Prostate cancer symptoms—when they do occur—are similar to symptoms of enlarged prostate, often involving trouble with urinating (peeing). It can be difficult to tell the difference between the 2 conditions based on symptoms alone. Symptoms of both include:

- Difficulty starting the flow of urine
- Weak or slow urine stream
- Feeling like your bladder is never fully empty
- Sudden urge to urinate
- Having to urinate too often, particularly at night

BPH doesn't cause prostate cancer and it doesn't turn into prostate cancer. But it's important to know that you can have BPH and **also** have prostate cancer.

Where does the prostate fit in?

The prostate is a gland located in the pelvis—the area between your hips. The prostate is important for sexual reproduction.

Prostate: A gland in the male reproductive system. A gland is an organ that makes fluids or chemicals the body needs. The prostate gland makes a protein (prostate-specific antigen, or PSA) that nourishes and helps transmit semen. The prostate also contains muscles that help propel semen through the urethra during ejaculation.

Semen: Fluid made up of liquids from the prostate and the seminal vesicles as well as sperm from the testicles. During ejaculation, semen is released from the body through the urethra and out through the penis.

Urethra: A tube that carries urine from the bladder out of the body. The prostate surrounds the urethra just beneath the bladder.

Seminal vesicles: Two glands that make and store another part of the fluid that becomes semen. The seminal vesicles are located above the prostate and behind the bladder.

Bladder: The organ that holds urine.

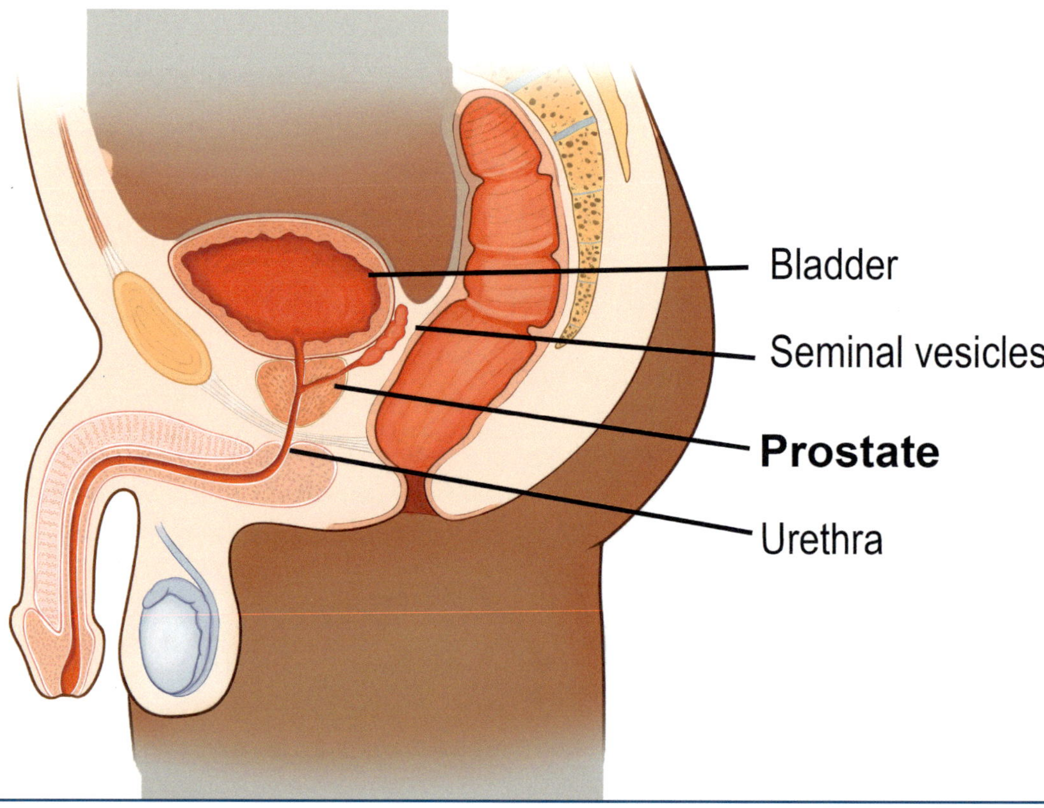

How did I get prostate cancer?

Cancer researchers don't know what causes prostate cells to grow out of control (become cancerous).

The fact is, everyone with a prostate has a risk for getting prostate cancer. This includes males as well as transgender females.

Several factors are linked to a higher risk for prostate cancer. These are called risk factors. A risk factor is anything that increases your chance of getting cancer. Risk factors don't necessarily cause prostate cancer, but people with prostate cancer usually have one or more of these risk factors:

Age

The biggest risk factor for prostate cancer is age. Prostate cancer is diagnosed most often in people aged 65 years and above. Your chances of getting prostate cancer increase as you become older.

Family history

Your family health history is information about the diseases and health conditions that have occurred in your family. A family history can reflect a pattern of certain diseases among family members. Having a close family member with prostate cancer (a sibling or parent) means you have a greater chance of getting it yourself.

People with a family history of certain cancers (breast, ovarian, colon, pancreatic, and others) may also be at a higher risk for prostate cancer.

Genetic factors

If cancer occurs often in your family, genetic testing can be done to find specific genetic changes known to be linked with prostate cancer and other cancers. For instance, having an inherited genetic change in the *BRCA1* or *BRCA2* gene increases your risk for prostate cancer as well as your risk for cancer that grows more quickly.

Race

In the United States, Black males are more likely than white males to develop prostate cancer. Prostate cancer in Black males is also more likely to occur at an earlier age and be more aggressive and more advanced when diagnosed. Black males are also twice as likely to die of prostate cancer than white males.

Several things contribute to these differences, such as barriers to accessing health care (including early detection screening), biological and genetic factors, and other causes. Researchers are trying to understand the reasons for these differences and what can be done to improve outcomes.

In light of these issues, Black males are encouraged to talk with their doctors or other health care providers about getting screening tests earlier and perhaps more often than what's recommended for those at average risk.

Diet and lifestyle

No diet has been found to cause prostate cancer or to prevent it. However, eating foods high in fat, such as meat and dairy products, has been linked to an increased risk for prostate cancer. Smoking also increases the risks for developing and dying from prostate cancer.

On the other hand, people who eat more fruits and vegetables have a lower risk for developing prostate cancer. Maintaining a healthy body weight through diet and exercise may slow the growth of prostate cancer and lower your risk for dying of it.

> **“The start of a cancer diagnosis feels a lot like beginning to climb a mountain: It’s unfamiliar terrain and you can’t see the summit. It’s important to take things one day at a time. Break everything down into bite-sized pieces and don’t expend emotional energy on the things you can’t control.”**

Key points

- Everyone with a prostate is at risk for prostate cancer.
- For most people, prostate cancer usually grows slowly and stays within the prostate.
- Most people with early-stage prostate cancer don’t have symptoms. And not everyone diagnosed with prostate cancer needs treatment.
- Age is the leading risk factor for prostate cancer. As you age, your chances of developing prostate cancer increase.
- People with a family history of certain other cancers may also be at a higher risk for prostate cancer.

Questions to ask

- If I don’t have any symptoms, do I need any treatment?
- Is my prostate cancer hereditary?
- How does having a relative with prostate, breast, or ovarian cancer increase my risk for prostate cancer?
- What are the chances the cancer has already spread from my prostate to another part of my body?
- Does this hospital or cancer center offer the best treatment for me?

3

Testing for early-stage prostate cancer

Several tests are needed to diagnose prostate cancer and to learn whether it's early- or advanced-stage cancer. The results of these tests will help your doctors and care team plan the best treatment for you.

About testing

Health care providers use a variety of tests to find prostate cancer and to determine how advanced the cancer is.

Tests are used to plan treatment, check how well treatment is working, and monitor your health after treatment ends.

This chapter will help you know what tests you might have and what to expect during testing. Not every person with prostate cancer will receive every test listed here. See **Guide 1**.

Common prostate tests

Common prostate cancer tests are used to detect the likelihood of prostate cancer in someone who has no symptoms, which is most often the case.

These tests are also used in people who have been diagnosed with prostate cancer to monitor their cancer and to check whether their treatment is working.

These 2 tests are the prostate-specific antigen (PSA) test and the digital rectal exam.

PSA test

This is a blood test that measures the amount of PSA in your bloodstream. PSA is a protein made inside of the prostate gland. Its job is to help semen transport sperm. While most PSA goes into semen, a little bit ends up in the bloodstream, too.

Guide 1
Possible tests for early-stage prostate cancer

Common prostate tests

- PSA test
- Digital rectal exam

General health tests

- Health history
- Family history
- Symptoms and quality of life assessment
- Blood and urine tests

Imaging tests

- MRI scan
- CT scan
- PET scan (PET/CT, PET/MRI)
- Bone scan

Biopsy

Biomarker and genetic tests

- Biomarker test
- Genetic test for inherited risk

All prostate cells, both normal cells and cancer cells, make PSA. If there's something wrong with the prostate—such as prostate cancer—the prostate can release more PSA into the bloodstream. An unusually high amount of PSA in the blood may be a sign of prostate cancer. Likewise, an increase in PSA after treatment may indicate the treatment is losing effectiveness.

However, age and other factors—such as an enlarged prostate or a urinary tract infection—can also cause high levels of PSA.

This means that a PSA test by itself can't provide a diagnosis of prostate cancer. That's why PSA testing is often paired with imaging or a digital rectal exam, or both, to decide whether you need a biopsy.

PSA level (also called total PSA) is measured in nanograms of PSA per milliliter (ng/mL) of blood.

> **"Be your own advocate. Talk to someone who has gone through the same thing as you. Ask a lot of questions, even the ones you are afraid to ask. You have to protect yourself and ensure you make the best decisions for you, and get the best care for your particular situation."**

Digital rectal exam

Don't be fooled by the name—no high-tech electronics are used in a digital rectal exam. For this test, the word digital refers to a finger (digit). The doctor will insert a gloved and

PSA testing

Prostate-specific antigen (PSA) is a protein made in the prostate gland. If there's something wrong with the prostate, it can release more PSA. An unusually high amount of PSA in the blood may be a sign of prostate cancer.

But a high PSA level doesn't automatically mean you have prostate cancer. Rather, it's a warning sign that you may need further testing.

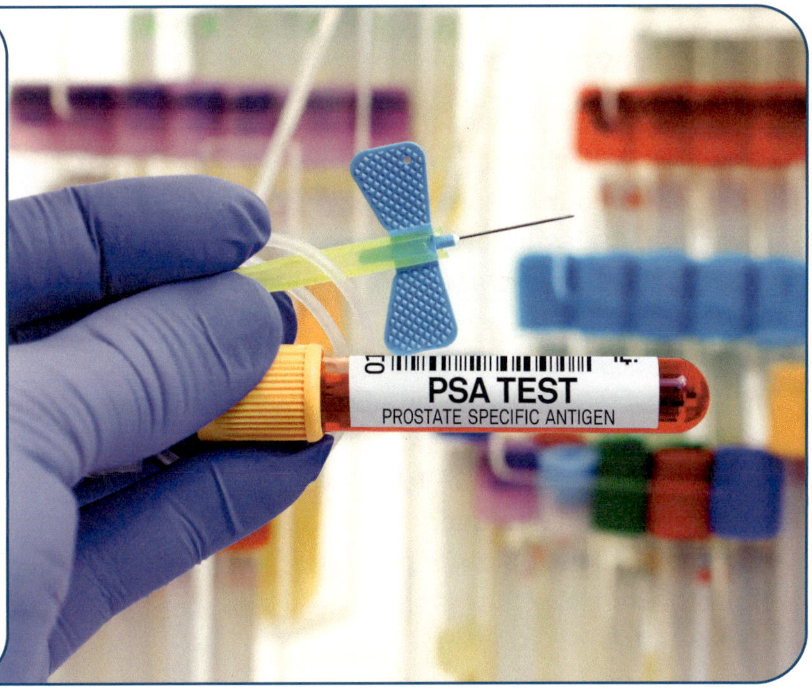

lubricated finger into your rectum to feel your prostate for any signs of cancer. An irregular or hardened part of the prostate could be a sign of a tumor.

A digital rectal exam (also called a prostate exam) may be an awkward and unpleasant form of testing. But it's the simplest and most direct way to check the size and texture of your prostate.

Not all parts of the prostate can be felt during a digital rectal exam, though. So it's usually paired with a PSA test and other factors—your age, race, family history, and more—to determine whether you need further testing.

Some doctors don't recommend a digital rectal exam because it's not very good at finding cancer on its own. So your doctor might leave the choice whether to have it up to you. NCCN experts say a digital rectal exam is most useful for individuals who have a higher PSA level.

Don't fear the digital rectal exam

A digital rectal exam is the simplest and most direct way to check the size and texture of your prostate. Although it can be uncomfortable, it's over in less than a minute.

General health tests

Health history

Your care team needs to have all of your health information. They'll ask you about any health problems and treatments you've had in your life. Be prepared to talk about any illness or injury you've had and when it happened.

Digital rectal exam

A digital rectal exam is a procedure in which your doctor inserts a finger into your rectum to feel your prostate. An irregular or hardened part of the prostate could be a sign of a tumor.

Not all parts of the prostate can be felt during this exam, though. So other tests, like PSA level and imaging scans, are used to get a more complete picture of your prostate health.

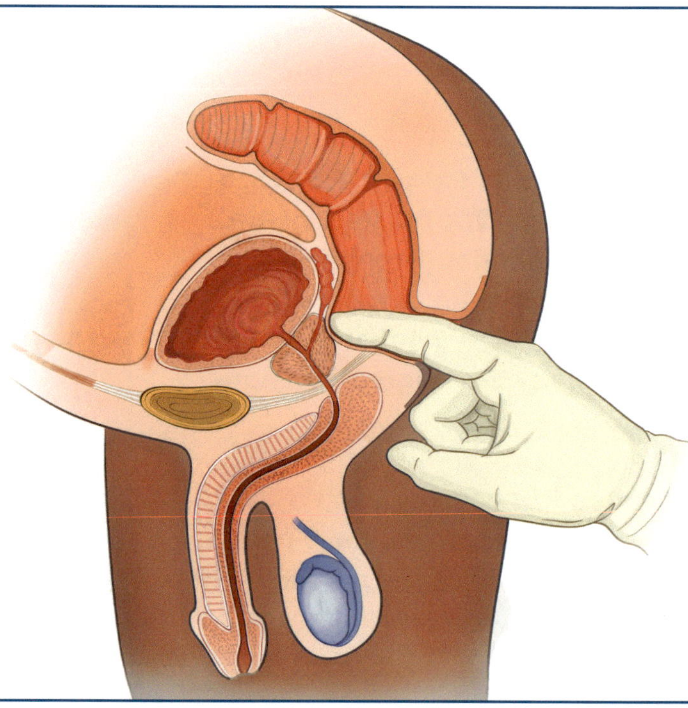

Also tell your care team about any symptoms you have.

Bring a list of your regular medicines and any over-the-counter medicines, herbals, or supplements you take. Some of these (such as saw palmetto, St. John's wort, or finasteride [Propecia] for hair loss) can cause changes in your PSA level, so your health care team needs to know if you're taking them.

Family history

Some cancers and other diseases can run in families. Your care team will ask about the health history of family members who are blood relatives. This information is called a family history.

It's important to ask members from both sides of your family about all cancers, not just prostate cancer. Ask family members if any relatives had cancer, at what age they were diagnosed, and if they died of it.

Also ask family members about other health issues like heart disease, stroke, and diabetes. Share this information and any changes in your family history with your care team.

Symptoms and quality of life

Your doctor or another member of your care team will ask you a series of questions about what symptoms you may have (such as peeing frequently, difficulty peeing or pooping, or sexual problems). You'll also be asked how these symptoms affect your quality of life.

Quality of life refers to your overall satisfaction with your well-being and your ability to participate in regular activities. It's important to answer all these questions honestly and completely so your care team has a full and up-to-date assessment of how you're doing.

Blood and urine tests

For a blood test, a needle is inserted into a vein in your arm to remove a sample of

When you go to health care visits, bring someone with you to listen, ask questions, and write down the answers.

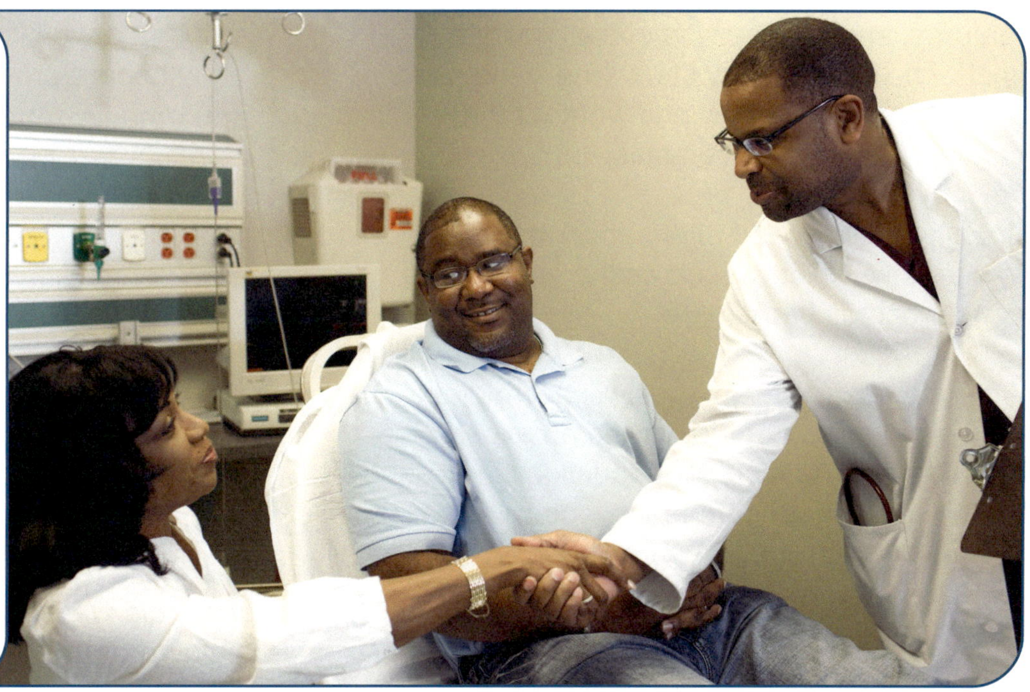

blood. The sample is examined in a lab where cells, proteins, and other components of the blood are tested for signs of disease or other conditions.

If your PSA level is high, you may need additional blood or urine testing.

Diagnostic tests

If the PSA test, digital rectal exam, blood or urine tests, or other factors (like family history, race, or age) suggest you may have prostate cancer, you'll be offered diagnostic testing. Diagnostic tests are used to confirm you have cancer.

Diagnostic tests include imaging scans, biopsies, and genetic tests.

Imaging tests

An imaging test takes pictures (images) of the inside of your body. The images can reveal cancer, including its size, location, and other features, such as the size of the prostate itself. The images may show where the cancer started (primary tumor) and whether the cancer has spread (metastasized).

Imaging is also used after cancer treatment to see how well it worked and to check if the cancer comes back.

After the scan, your images will be studied by a radiologist. A radiologist is an expert at reading imaging tests. The radiologist will send the results to your care team, who will discuss the results with you. Be sure to ask any questions you may have.

Who's on your care team?

Treating prostate cancer takes a team approach. Some members of your care team will be with you throughout your treatment, while others will be there for parts of it.

Your team should communicate and work together to bring the best knowledge from each specialty.

Lead members of your team should include prostate cancer specialists, such as a urologist, radiation oncologist, and medical oncologist.

Other common team members include your primary care doctor, nurse, physical therapist, physician assistant, mental health care provider, genetic counselor, pharmacist, patient navigator, social worker, sex therapist, and nutritionist or dietitian.

Imaging methods for detecting prostate cancer include MRI, CT, PET, bone scan, or a combination of these.

MRI scan

A magnetic resonance imaging (MRI) scan uses radio waves and powerful magnets to provide a detailed view of the cancer within the prostate. It's also used to see if cancer has spread to nearby lymph nodes or to the bones in your pelvis.

An MRI scanner is a large machine with a tunnel in the middle. An MRI machine makes a lot of noise, but you can wear headphones or earplugs and listen to music.

An MRI scan of the prostate can help decide whether a biopsy is needed. MRI is frequently done before a biopsy to locate any suspicious areas in the prostate for the biopsy to target.

More commonly, MRI is used after diagnosis to learn whether the cancer has advanced outside of the prostate or into the lymph nodes. It can help to plan treatment or to decide whether active surveillance is appropriate. MRI can also be used after treatment to check if the cancer has come back (recurrence).

Because an MRI uses magnets, you can't bring any metal objects (such as a phone, jewelry, wristwatch, or belt with metal buckle) into the imaging room.

CT scan

If MRI is unavailable or not recommended for you, you might have a computed tomography (CT or CAT) scan instead. A CT scan takes many x-rays of your body from different angles. A computer combines the x-ray pictures to make a series of cross-sectional images of your pelvis.

A CT scan is most often used after diagnosis to determine the extent of cancer in your body (your cancer stage).

PET scan

A positron emission tomography (PET) scan highlights cells in your body that may be cancerous. A PET scan is done after you've been diagnosed to determine the extent of your cancer or to see if it has metastasized. PET imaging can also show how well treatment is working.

PET imaging

A positron emission tomography (PET) scan highlights cells in your body that may be cancerous. A PET scan is done after you've been diagnosed to determine the extent of your cancer or to see if it has metastasized. PET imaging can also show how well treatment is working.

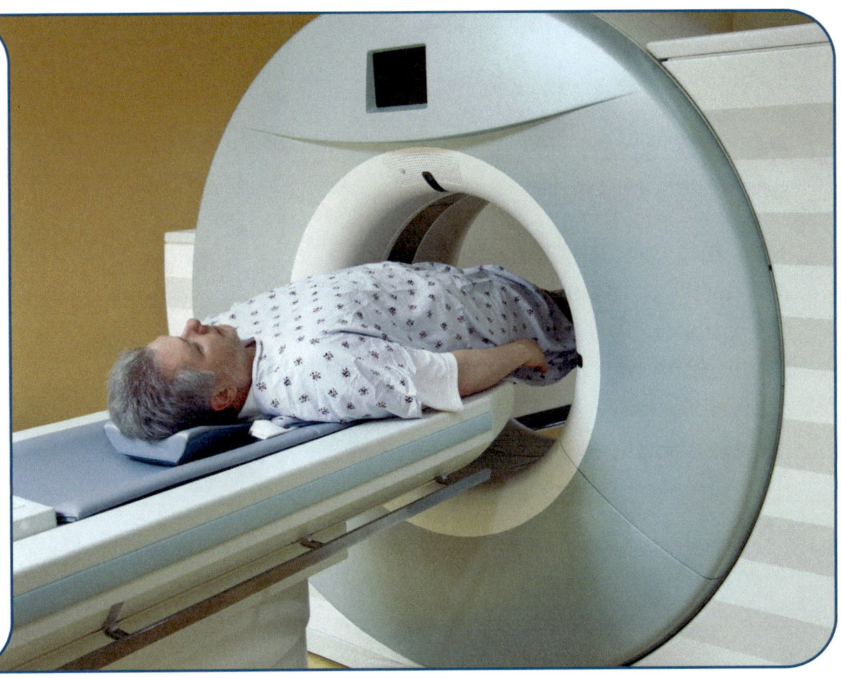

A PET scan requires injecting a radioactive substance called a tracer into your bloodstream. The tracer targets your cancer cells, which show up as bright spots on the scan.

Because PET uses a different imaging method, it's often combined with CT or MRI for an even more detailed image. These combined methods are called PET/CT and PET/MRI scans.

Bone scan

A bone scan can detect whether cancer has spread to your bones. A bone scan may be done if you have bone pain, a high risk for bone metastasis, or changes in certain test results. Bone scans may also be used to monitor how well treatment is working.

A bone scan uses a radioactive tracer to make pictures of the inside of bones. Before the pictures are taken, the tracer is injected into your bloodstream.

A special camera will take pictures of the tracer in your bones. Areas of bone damage absorb more tracer than healthy bone. Bone damage can be caused by cancer, cancer treatment, or other health problems. These damaged areas show up as bright spots on the scans.

Biopsy

Although a high PSA level and an abnormal digital rectal exam are signs of possible prostate cancer, the only way to confirm cancer is to have a biopsy.

A biopsy is a procedure in which a sample of cells or tissue is removed from your body and tested for cancer. You and your doctors will decide when, or if, you need a biopsy.

Your biopsy may be done in a surgical center under sedation or in your doctor's office with local anesthesia to numb the pain. If done in the office, you'll lie on your side with your knees curled up or on your back with your legs raised.

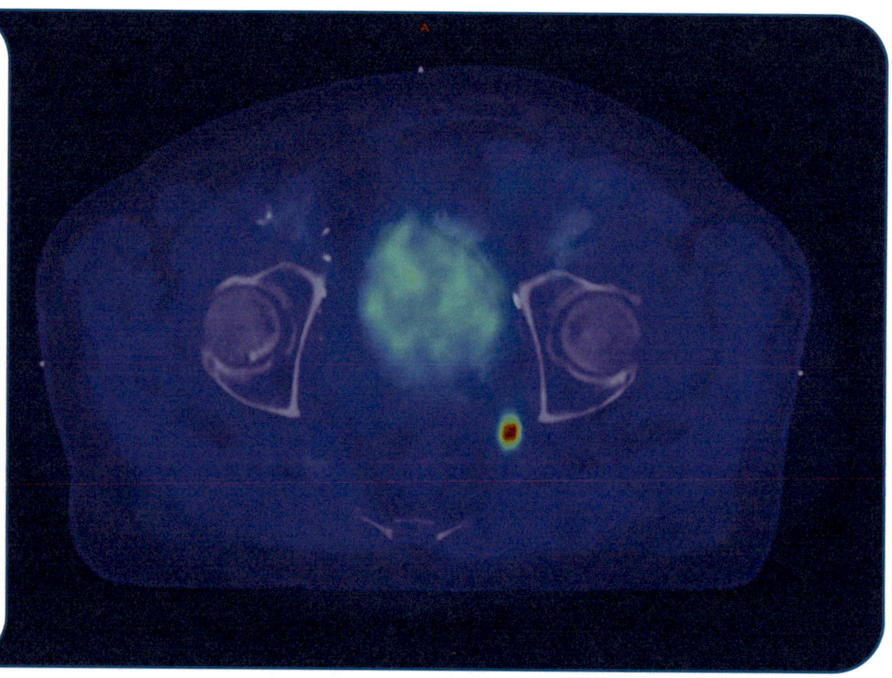

PET/CT scan of prostate cancer

This image combines PET and CT scans to show a cross-section of the pelvis. The greenish circle in the center of the image identifies cancer in the prostate, while the intense red dot indicates cancer that has spread to a pelvic lymph node.

Your doctor will insert a lubricated probe into your rectum. The probe provides ultrasound images that allow your care team to see your prostate inside your body. MRI scans of your prostate may be combined with the ultrasound images if your MRI before the biopsy showed any concerning lesions.

Using ultrasound (with or without MRI) for guidance, your doctor will insert a hollow needle either through the rectum or through the perineum (the skin between the anus and scrotum) and into the prostate gland.

When the needle is removed, it will pull out a small sample of prostate tissue called a core. A core sample is only about the size of a grain of rice.

Your doctor will usually take at least 12 core samples from various parts of the prostate as well as several targeted samples from suspicious areas of the prostate identified on the MRI. Checking different areas provides a more complete evaluation of cancer throughout the gland.

After the biopsy samples are removed, a specialist called a pathologist will examine the samples under a microscope and test them for cancer cells. The pathologist will find out how many of the core samples contain cancer and will also measure the percentage of cancer in each core.

With this information, the pathologist can estimate the amount of cancer in the prostate and how aggressive it may be. Also, by identifying where each core sample was taken, your team will know if the cancer is concentrated in a certain section of the prostate.

The pathologist will put these results into a report. Ask your doctor or another member of your care team to review the pathology report with you.

Biopsy of the prostate

A biopsy removes a sample of tissue that is tested for cancer. Shown here is a transperineal biopsy, in which a needle is inserted through the perineum and into the prostate. An ultrasound probe, which goes into the rectum, helps the doctor guide the needle into the prostate. MRI scans of your prostate may be combined with the ultrasound image to provide a highly accurate picture of the cancer.

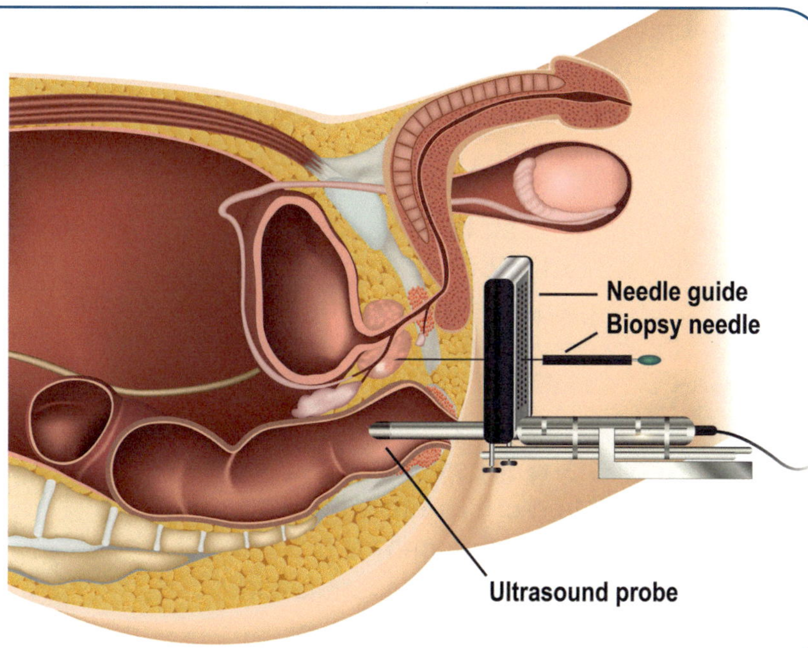

It's common to have more than one biopsy if you're on active surveillance. You'll have one biopsy to determine your diagnosis and often another biopsy within a year (called a confirmatory biopsy) to see if any changes have happened over time.

Most biopsies are safe, but sometimes they can cause complications. Complications can include infection, bleeding from the rectum, or blood in the urine, stool, or semen. These usually go away after a few days. Blood in the semen may take longer to go away.

It's also important to know that a biopsy won't cause prostate cancer to spread or worsen.

Biomarker test

A biomarker is something found in your body that can be measured to provide information about your health.

In cancer care, a biomarker is a characteristic that can be used to identify certain cancer cells. Therapy that targets such characteristics can find and destroy those cells. For example, certain mutations (changes) in the tumor's DNA are biomarkers, which can be targeted with specific treatments. Biomarker testing looks for such changes.

Biomarker testing—also called tumor mutation testing or tumor profiling—is typically performed on a piece of tumor tissue removed during a biopsy or surgery, or on a sample of your blood.

Importantly, biomarker testing can help guide treatment. It can find out whether someone's cancer has a mutation that can be treated with therapy that targets that specific mutation.

“

It's important to know that a biopsy won't cause prostate cancer to spread or worsen.”

Biomarker testing can also provide clues about whether the cancer is at a lower or higher risk for growing and spreading. If the cancer is low risk, you may be able to put off treatment, which also avoids treatment-related complications and side effects. If the cancer is high risk, your doctor may recommend starting treatment soon.

Biomarker testing is different from hereditary genetic testing. Biomarker testing looks for somatic mutations in genes. Somatic (or acquired) mutations happened in your lifetime and can't be passed down in families.

Ask your care team if biomarker testing is right for you.

Genetic test for inherited risk

Genetic testing looks for germline (inherited) mutations, which are passed from parents to children.

Most prostate cancers are not hereditary. But if you have a family history of certain cancers or you have higher-risk prostate cancer, your doctor might suggest genetic testing to find out if you have a germline (inherited) cancer risk.

Your doctor can talk to you about testing or refer you to a genetic counselor. This is an expert who has special training in genetic diseases. A genetic counselor can help you decide whether you're a good candidate for genetic testing, including whether your risk is high enough to make genetic testing worthwhile. If you have genetic testing, a genetic counselor can interpret the results for you.

For more information on genetic testing for hereditary prostate cancer, see *NCCN Guidelines for Patients: Genetic Testing for Hereditary Breast, Ovarian, Pancreatic, and Prostate Cancers*, available at NCCN.org/patientguidelines and on the NCCN Patient Guides for Cancer app.

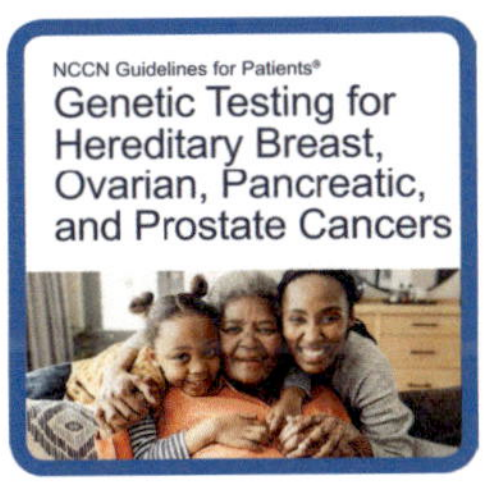

Key points

- A high or rising amount of prostate-specific antigen (PSA) in the bloodstream may be a sign of prostate cancer.
- A digital rectal exam is the simplest way to check the size and texture of your prostate.
- A biopsy is used to confirm (diagnose) prostate cancer. It's a procedure that removes samples of cells or tissue to find cancer.
- Imaging tests may be done to see if the cancer has spread beyond the prostate.
- An MRI scan of the prostate can help decide whether a biopsy is needed.
- A genetic test is used to find out if you have an inherited risk for cancer.
- Biomarker testing looks for specific changes that can be used to identify certain cancer cells. Some of these biomarkers may be targeted for treatment.

Questions to ask

- What tests will I have? How do I prepare for testing?
- Do the tests have any risks?
- Will any of the tests hurt?
- What are the advantages and disadvantages of having genetic testing?
- How soon will I know my test results and who will explain them to me?

What's next?

You've had numerous tests to find out if you have prostate cancer. Next, your care team will use your test results to figure out whether the cancer is at a lower risk or higher risk.

Once your level of risk has been identified, your team will assess whether you need treatment and, if so, what your treatment plan will be.

4

Assessing your risk

It's important to know the risk for your cancer getting worse. Your care team will look at key features of the cancer to assess this risk. This chapter explains each of these characteristics.

After being told you have cancer, your next thought may be, "How soon should I start treatment to get rid of it?"

The fact is, a lot of people with early-stage prostate cancer don't need treatment right away. Many never need treatment.

To determine when you should start treatment, your doctor or care team will conduct a risk assessment. This involves determining how likely the cancer is to remain within the prostate or to spread outside of the prostate.

A risk assessment also considers whether the cancer may come back after treatment (recurrence) and, if so, whether it can be controlled with a different type of treatment.

To assess risk, your care providers use these tools: **Risk groups**, **Life expectancy**, **Nomograms**, and **Specialized risk tests**. Let's look at each of these assessment tools in turn.

Risk groups

Why do you need to know your risk group? Because your risk group is the basis for your prognosis.

A prognosis predicts the likely course and outcome of a disease. Your prognosis guides your treatment options. For example, people with lower risk generally get minimal treatment or no treatment at all. People with higher risk usually have more aggressive treatment.

Anyone who has a prostate is at risk for prostate cancer. But your chances of getting prostate cancer increase as you grow older.

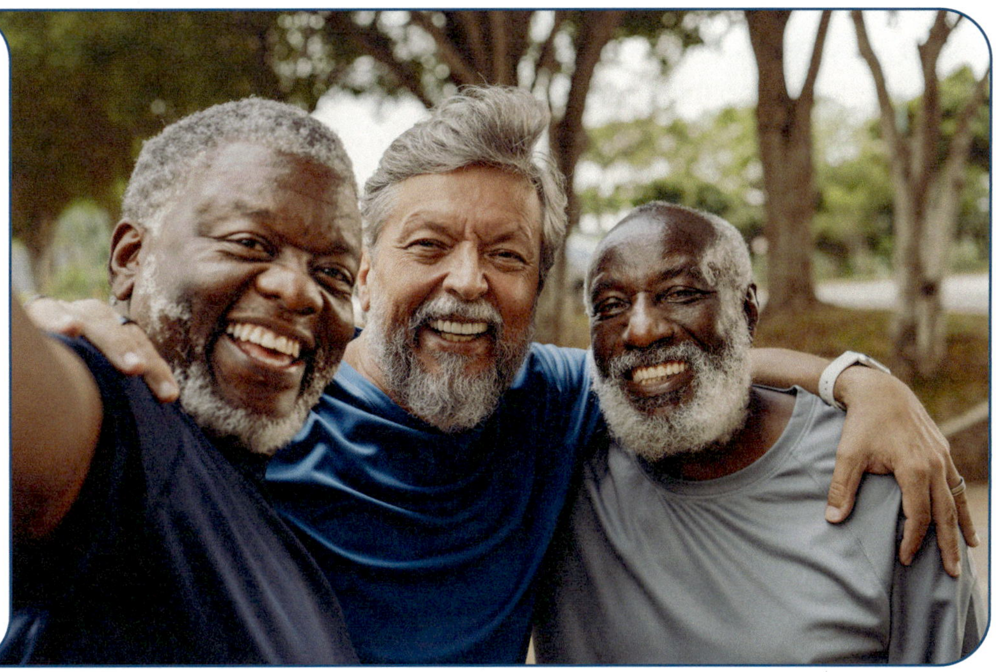

> **“**
> **It’s OK to have bad days, but don’t let yourself stay there. A positive attitude goes a long way.”**

Your disease will be classified into 1 of 5 different risk groups, from low risk to very high risk. Your risk group will be based on the clinical features of your cancer: PSA level, Grade Group, tumor stage, and biopsy results.

PSA level

A simple blood test will tell you how much prostate-specific antigen (PSA) is in your bloodstream. A high PSA level may indicate a risk for prostate cancer. However, high PSA levels can vary by age, race, and other factors.

- **Age** – PSA level tends to increase with age. For people in their 40s, a PSA level above 2.5 ng/mL may be suspicious for prostate cancer. For those in their 50s and over, 3.0 ng/mL or higher can be suspicious. A PSA level of 10 ng/mL or higher is a danger sign at any age.
- **Race** – Normal PSA levels tend to be higher in Black males than in white males—about 1 point higher on average among males of the same age. Researchers don’t know the reason for this difference, but they’re investigating it.
- **Enlarged prostate** – The larger the prostate, the more PSA it can make. Other health issues besides cancer can also cause an enlarged prostate.
- **Sex and exercise** – PSA may increase after ejaculation or vigorous exercise. Your doctor may recommend avoiding sex and exercise for 1 or 2 days before a PSA test. This short break allows PSA to return to its usual level.
- **Drugs and supplements** – Some medicines, herbals, and supplements can also affect PSA level.
- **Biopsy** – PSA level rises temporarily after a biopsy of the prostate.

PSA level doesn’t tell the whole story, though. There are other ways that PSA can be interpreted, such as PSA density.

PSA density

If you have a larger prostate, you’re also likely to have a higher PSA level. But that doesn’t mean you have a greater risk for prostate cancer. Likewise, people with small or very small prostates and low PSA levels aren’t necessarily at lower risk.

To adjust for this, your care team can calculate PSA density.

PSA density is the amount of PSA compared to the size of the prostate. A higher PSA density indicates a greater likelihood of cancer.

Grade Group

If cancer cells are found in your biopsy samples, further testing can identify your cancer risk.

Results from these tests may indicate that the cancer will grow and spread quickly, for example. Or the results may suggest that the cancer will grow very slowly and not spread outside of the prostate at all. This information helps plan the best treatment for your type of cancer.

By looking at your biopsy samples, the pathologist will identify certain cancer cell patterns (called Gleason patterns), which are used to calculate your Gleason score. This translates to your Grade Group:

Gleason patterns

↓

Gleason score

↓

Grade Group

Your Grade Group is combined with other factors to determine your risk group.

This can be confusing at first, but it's not all that complicated in the end. Read on.

Gleason patterns

After studying your biopsy sample under a microscope, the pathologist will assign a number based on the pattern of cancer cells (Gleason pattern) in the sample.

A pattern that looks more like normal cells is given a lower number. A cell pattern that looks more abnormal is assigned a higher number.

Gleason patterns range from 1 to 5. However, patterns 1 and 2 are not considered cancer and are no longer used. So the lowest is pattern 3, which looks the most like normal cells.

Gleason score

If prostate tumors contained only one pattern of cancer cells, estimating risk would be much easier. But prostate tumors often contain more than one pattern of cells.

To account for this, the 2 most common Gleason patterns found in the biopsy sample are combined into a single Gleason score. The pattern of cancer cells that takes up the largest area in the sample is assigned the first number. The pattern that accounts for the second largest area is given the second number.

These 2 numbers added together results in a Gleason score. For example:

pattern 3 + pattern 4 =

Gleason score of 7

A Gleason score represents how much your biopsy sample looks like normal prostate tissue. It also estimates how aggressive your prostate cancer is—that is, how quickly it might grow and whether it will spread. A higher Gleason score means the cancer is more likely to grow and spread quickly than cancer with a lower Gleason score.

Gleason scores range from 6 to 10, where 6 is the lowest score. A Gleason score of 7 is intermediate grade, and 8 to 10 is high grade. This can be confusing because 6 seems like it would be a medium score, not a low score. So, to make Gleason scores simpler to use, they can be converted into Grade Groups.

Grade Groups

A Grade Group is a way to interpret a Gleason score. There are 5 Grade Groups, numbered 1 to 5. The higher the Grade Group, the more aggressive the cancer. So cancer with a Gleason score of 6, the lowest score, is equal to Grade Group 1. Likewise, cancer with a Gleason score of 9 or 10 becomes Grade Group 5, the highest score.

Guide 2
How to find your risk from your Gleason score

Gleason patterns	Gleason score	Grade Group	Prognosis
3+3	6	1	**Low-grade cancer** is less aggressive and is likely to grow and spread very slowly. If the cancer is small, many years may pass before it becomes a problem. Low-grade cancer may never need treatment.
3+4	7	2	**Intermediate-grade cancer** is moderately aggressive and is likely to grow and spread at a modest pace. If the cancer is small, several years may pass before it becomes a problem. To prevent problems, treatment may be needed.
4+3	7	3	
4+4 3+5 5+3	8	4	**High-grade cancer** is very aggressive and is likely to grow and spread quickly. If the cancer is small, a few years may pass before the cancer becomes a life-threatening problem. But to prevent problems, treatment is needed now.
4+5 5+4 5+5	9 or 10	5	

Grade Group 1 indicates low risk. Grade Groups 2 and 3 correspond to intermediate risk. Grade Groups 4 and 5 predict high risk and very high risk. See **Guide 2**.

Importantly, Grade Group also takes into account that Groups 2 and 3 are different even though each one has a Gleason score of 7. The difference is the cancer in Grade Group 3 is more serious. Why? Because the first number of the Gleason score in Grade Group 3 (**4**+3) is higher than the first number in Grade Group 2 (**3**+4). Remember, the first number is given to the cancer pattern that makes up the largest area of the biopsy sample.

Tumor stage

The next characteristic that contributes to your overall risk group is the tumor stage.

Staging is a way to describe how much cancer is in your body and whether it has spread. Knowing your stage is important for predicting the course of your disease and for making a treatment plan.

The tumor, node, metastasis (TNM) system is used to stage prostate cancer. In this system, the letters T, N, and M stand for different areas of cancer growth:

- **T (tumor)** – Describes the size of the main (primary) tumor and if it has grown outside of the prostate
- **N (node)** – Identifies whether cancer has spread to the lymph nodes
- **M (metastasis)** – Indicates if cancer has spread to distant parts of the body (metastasized)

Your doctor will assign a number to each letter, based on your test results. For example, the number after T ranges from 1 through 4 based on the tumor's size and growth. The larger the tumor or the more the cancer has spread, the higher the number. A zero (0) after T means there is no tumor.

The T, N, and M scores are combined to assign a **stage** to the cancer.

Let's say your prostate cancer is given a TNM score of T2, N0, M0. This score means that the tumor is big enough to be felt during a digital rectal exam (T2). But the numbers after N and M are zeros because early-stage cancer hasn't spread outside the prostate gland to lymph nodes (N0) or to distant parts of the body (M0).

A letter may also be included after the tumor stage (T2a, for example) to give more information based on the digital rectal exam or an examination of prostate tissue. The letter stands for the extent of cancer and/or its location in the prostate. See **Guide 3**.

Cancer staging is often done twice. The first time is before any treatment. The second time is during or after treatment to see how well the treatment has worked.

Biopsy results

Results from your core needle biopsy also help to determine your overall risk group. One finding is the number of core samples that contain cancer (for example, 5 out of 12 in each core).

Using this information, the pathologist can estimate the amount of cancer in the entire prostate.

Biopsy results can also show whether the cancer is concentrated in a certain section (or sections) of the prostate.

Guide 3
Tumor details for T stage

T1 – The tumor can't be felt by a digital rectal exam, but a biopsy found cancer cells	**T1a**	The tumor is found unexpectedly during another procedure. Only a small part (5 percent [5%] or less) of the removed tissue is cancer.
	T1b	The tumor is found unexpectedly during another procedure. More than a small part (more than 5 percent [5%]) of the removed tissue is cancer.
	T1c	PSA level is high and calls for a biopsy of the prostate.
T2 – The tumor can be felt by a digital rectal exam but it hasn't spread outside the prostate	**T2a**	Cancer is found in half or less than half of one side of the prostate.
	T2b	Cancer is found in more than half of one side of the prostate, but it isn't in both sides.
	T2c	Cancer has grown into both sides of the prostate.
T3 – The tumor has spread outside the prostate to nearby tissues, but no farther	**T3a**	Cancer has grown outside the prostate, but not into the seminal vesicle(s).
	T3b	Cancer has grown outside the prostate and into the seminal vesicle(s).
T4 – The tumor has spread outside the prostate to nearby tissues and also to other areas	**T4**	Cancer has grown outside the prostate and spread to nearby tissues or organs, such as the bladder, rectum, pelvic wall, and/or pelvic muscles

What's your risk group?

Based on the results of these tests and calculations—PSA level, Grade Group, tumor stage, and biopsy results—you'll be placed into an initial risk group. See **Guide 4**.

Your risk group helps determine which treatment options may be best for you. Using these tests together to create risk groups is more reliable than using any test by itself to choose treatment options.

Guide 4
Characteristics that make up your risk group

Risk group	PSA level	Grade Group	Tumor stage	Biopsy results
Low risk	Must have **all** of these characteristics			
	Less than 10 ng/mL	1	T1 to T2a	
Favorable intermediate risk	**Only 1** of these characteristics needed			**And** cancer found in fewer than half of all biopsy cores
	10 to 20 ng/mL	2	T2b or T2c	
Unfavorable intermediate risk	Must have **2 or 3** of these characteristics			**Or at least 1** of these characteristics **and** cancer found in more than half of all biopsy cores
	10 to 20 ng/mL	2 or 3	T2b or T2c	
High risk	Must have **at least 1** of these characteristics			
	More than 20 ng/mL	4 or 5	T3a to T4	
Very high risk	Must have **at least 2** of these characteristics			
	More than 40 ng/mL	4 or 5	T3 to T4	

But risk groups aren't the only risk assessment tool. There's also life expectancy, nomograms, and specialized risk tests.

Life expectancy

Life expectancy is the average lifespan of a person. It's measured in years. An estimate of your life expectancy is a key factor in deciding which tests and treatments you'll need.

It's important to know that life expectancy—when used for cancer care—is an estimate based on large numbers of people. That means life expectancy can be applied to a certain population or age range, but it's not as easy to make a precise estimate of the lifespan of an individual person.

So why estimate your life expectancy? Sometimes, patients in certain risk groups should wait until symptoms appear before having tests or starting treatment. There may be no benefit to having additional tests or undergoing treatment if you don't have any symptoms or if you have other more life-threatening health conditions.

If you don't have any symptoms and you have low-risk or intermediate-risk prostate cancer with an estimated life expectancy of 5 to 10 years, then observation is usually recommended. Observation is different from active surveillance, which usually involves routine imaging and biopsies.

We'll talk more about life expectancy and how it impacts treatment options in Chapter *5: Types of treatment.*

Nomograms

A nomogram predicts your prognosis, which is the likely course your cancer will take. A nomogram uses math to compare you and your prostate cancer to hundreds or thousands of other people who have been treated for prostate cancer.

Your doctor can use a nomogram to predict how likely your cancer is to grow or spread, based on your test results.

Risk groups and nomograms both provide information that is specific to you, but nomograms can give slightly more accurate estimates of cancer risk. Both are used, along with other risk assessment tools, to plan treatment.

Specialized risk tests

Your doctor or health care provider can order tests to help better understand how aggressive your cancer is.

One of these tests looks at the molecular characteristics and gene expression (which genes are turned on) in a sample of your tumor.

Another test looks at a digital image of your cancer biopsy and uses artificial intelligence to predict potential treatment.

Depending on your situation, results from these tests may help identify the right treatment for you and avoid under-treatment or over-treatment.

These tests don't replace standard measures, such as PSA, Gleason score, Grade Group, and imaging. They're used in addition to them.

If you have any questions about why you're having a test or what it means, ask your doctor or care team.

Key points

- A risk assessment determines how likely the cancer is to remain within the prostate or to spread outside of the prostate.
- People with lower risk generally get minimal or no active treatment. People with higher risk usually get more aggressive treatment.
- Cancer staging describes how much cancer is in the body and where it's located.
- Life expectancy is an estimate of the number of years you will likely live. It's based on large numbers of people and is not an exact prediction. But it can help choose the best treatment for you.
- A nomogram predicts the course your cancer will likely take (prognosis).
- Specialized risk tests may help identify the right treatment for you and avoid under-treatment or over-treatment.

Questions to ask

- What's the risk that my cancer will grow and spread outside of my prostate gland?
- Can you explain how estimated life expectancy is different from how long I might actually live?
- How do my age, race, overall health, and other factors affect my options?
- Will I need PSA tests, digital rectal exams, and biopsies for the rest of my life?

What's next?

This chapter explained how your health care team figures out the risk for your prostate cancer to grow and spread. Your risk level determines which treatments you can get. Early-stage cancer grows slowly and may not spread. So you might not need treatment right away.

Still, it's important to know about all your treatment options. The next chapter describes each treatment for early-stage prostate cancer. After that, you'll learn which treatments may work best for your level of risk.

5

Types of treatment

There's more than one treatment for prostate cancer. This chapter describes the many treatment options. Talk with your care team about which treatment might be best for you.

Prostate cancer is usually a slow-growing disease. It's also a complex disease with many treatment options. Common treatments for early-stage prostate cancer include surgery and radiation therapy, which are sometimes combined with hormone therapy.

Or, your treatment plan may include no direct therapy but instead involve active surveillance or observation.

> **"When you are deciding on your treatment options, remember that even though some decisions need to be made fast, don't rush. Think through your options and get second, or even third, opinions. Have people you can trust to talk through your options, so you feel comfortable in your decisions."**

Active surveillance

Active surveillance is a plan that closely watches your condition, with treatment at the ready if needed.

Because a small tumor can grow very slowly, it's possible to wait to treat prostate cancer until the tumor grows larger. During this time, you'll have tests and biopsies on a regular basis to look for changes in the tumor's growth.

Although your care team may ask you to have tests more or less frequently based on your risk, regular testing during active surveillance may follow a schedule something like this:

- Prostate-specific antigen (PSA) test twice a year
- Digital rectal exam once a year
- MRI scan every 1 to 2 years
- Prostate biopsy every 1 to 3 years or as needed

You won't receive any cancer treatment during active surveillance. But treatment will begin if your cancer grows or spreads.

Why wait to be treated? Mainly because surgery and other forms of treatment have side effects. If you can delay treatment without harm—or avoid it altogether—then you can also delay or entirely avoid the side effects of treatment. Side effects of surgery, radiation therapy, and other treatments can take a toll on your quality of life.

In general, active surveillance is the preferred strategy for people with lower-risk prostate cancer and a longer life expectancy. About half of these people are able to avoid treatment for 10 years or more.

To see if you're a good candidate for active surveillance, you may need a confirmatory MRI with or without a confirmatory prostate biopsy. These confirmatory tests are usually performed within a year of your diagnosis to see if there have been any changes during that time.

Other factors to consider for active surveillance:

- Your life expectancy
- Your overall health
- Features or unique qualities of your tumor
- Possible side effects of treatment
- Your wishes about treatment

A common question people have about active surveillance is: When do you know to switch from surveillance to treatment?

The main reason for switching is that your Grade Group went up after a recent biopsy. Additional reasons for starting treatment may include an increase in the size of the tumor or a rise in your PSA level.

Observation

Observation involves monitoring your prostate cancer and watching for symptoms. (You may hear it called watch-and-wait or watchful waiting.) If symptoms develop, treatment is often focused on palliative care or symptom relief instead of trying to cure the cancer.

Palliative care treats the symptoms of cancer and the side effects of cancer treatment. This allows patients to maintain a good quality of life without the burden of unnecessary treatment.

Observation often applies to individuals with intermediate-risk prostate cancer who are older or frail and have an estimated life expectancy of 5 to 10 years or less.

Observation is also recommended for individuals with low-risk prostate cancer and a short life expectancy (5 years or less). These people often have other health conditions that are more severe than their prostate cancer.

Observation is different from active surveillance. Observation is a less aggressive way to monitor prostate cancer. It doesn't require regular biopsies—just a visit for a physical and possibly a PSA test once or twice a year.

By comparison, active surveillance involves frequent testing to see whether the cancer is progressing. If it is, it can be treated before it gets worse.

Surgery

Surgery is a procedure to remove cancer from the body. The tumor is removed along with some normal-looking prostate tissue around its edge called the surgical margin.

- **A positive margin** is when cancer cells are found in the tissue that's removed with the tumor. The margin is "positive" for cancer.
- **A negative margin** is when no cancer cells are found in the tissue that's removed with the tumor. The margin is "negative" for cancer.

A negative margin is the better result because it means that all the tumor in that area has likely been removed. On the other hand, having a positive margin doesn't always mean that the cancer will grow back.

Surgery can be used as the main (primary) treatment. Or surgery may only be part of your treatment plan. The type of surgery you receive depends on the size and location of the tumor. It also depends on whether cancer is found in any surrounding organs or tissues.

Radical prostatectomy

Prostatectomy means removing the prostate gland through surgery. A radical prostatectomy removes not only the entire prostate but also the surrounding tissue, seminal vesicles, and sometimes the nearby lymph nodes.

Radical prostatectomy is often done when:

- The tumor has not grown outside of the prostate.
- The tumor can be removed completely with surgery.
- You have an estimated life expectancy of 10 years or more.
- You have no other serious health conditions.

A radical prostatectomy is complex and requires a great deal of skill. Surgeons experienced in this type of surgery often have better results.

There are 2 surgical methods for radical prostatectomy:

- **Open surgery** removes the prostate through a single cut or incision. The incision is long enough to let your doctor directly view and access the tumor to remove it.
- **Minimally invasive surgery** uses one or a few small incisions or holes instead of one larger cut. The surgeon inserts small tools through each incision to perform the surgery. In most centers, the surgeon uses a robot to guide the tools more precisely.

Minimally invasive surgery has become more common than open surgery. People who receive minimally invasive surgery may have shorter hospital stays, less blood loss, fewer surgical complications, and/or faster recovery time. However, the major side effects of minimally invasive radical prostatectomy—incontinence and erectile dysfunction—occur about as often as they do with open surgery.

Side effects of prostate surgery

Radical prostatectomy frequently causes 2 side effects: urinary incontinence and erectile dysfunction.

Urinary incontinence – After a radical prostatectomy, most people temporarily lose the ability to control when they pee. This is called urinary incontinence, and it can be a major problem.

Right after the procedure, a catheter will be inserted into your urethra to allow you to empty your bladder and for your urethra to heal. The catheter will stay in place for 1 to 2 weeks after surgery. You'll be shown how to care for it before you go home. If the catheter is removed too early, you may lose control of your bladder or be unable to urinate due to scar tissue.

After the catheter is removed, you may need to use absorbent pads or incontinence underwear for several weeks or months.

You can also do exercises to strengthen the pelvic floor muscle. If you haven't had prostate surgery yet, consider starting pelvic floor exercises beforehand to help to reduce urinary incontinence afterward.

In addition, certain prescription medications can reduce the need to pee so often.

Most patients gradually recover most of their bladder control within a year, though many continue to use pads for minor leaks. If incontinence continues to be a major problem, you can have a surgical procedure to help control urination.

Minimally invasive prostatectomy

A minimally invasive prostatectomy removes the prostate through one or more small keyhole incisions in the abdomen. In many centers, the surgeon performs the procedure using a robot. This provides greater precision and a highly magnified view of the prostate.

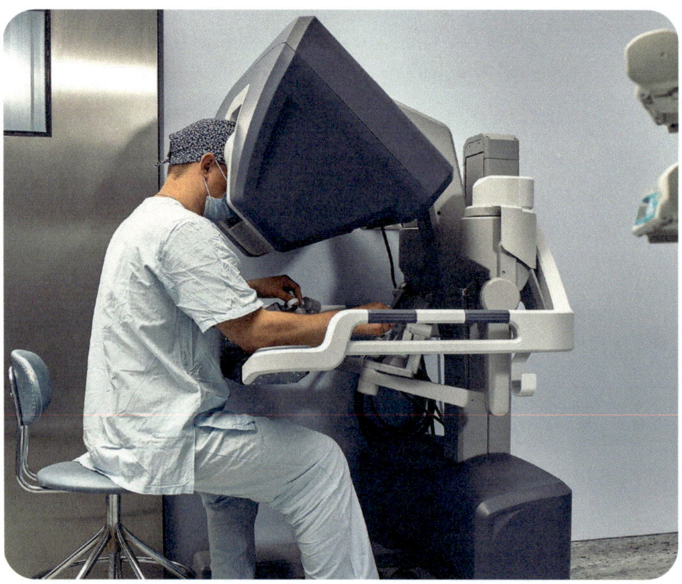

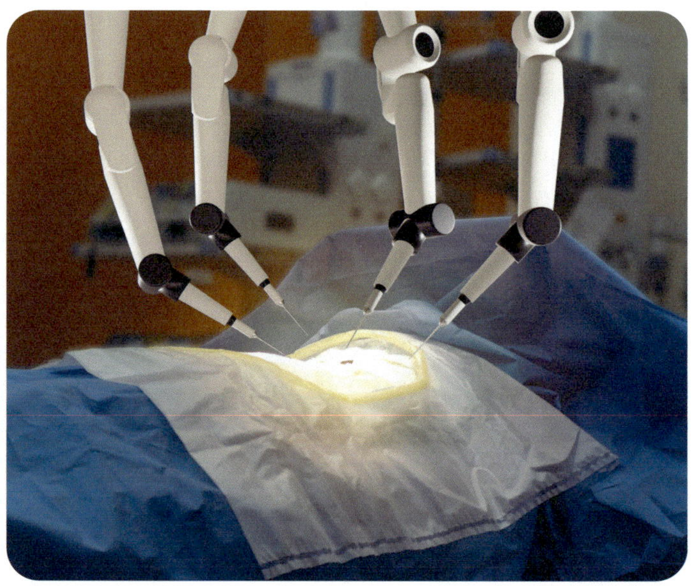

Erectile dysfunction – Erectile dysfunction means having difficulty or being unable to have an erection of the penis. It's a common problem after prostate surgery. But it often—although not always—improves over time.

Youll have higher risk for erectile dysfunction if:

- You are older
- You have erectile problems before surgery
- The nerves near your prostate are damaged or removed during surgery

The nerves near your prostate (called cavernous nerves) control the ability to have erections. Surgeons do their best to avoid these nerves when performing a prostatectomy, but damage to the nerves during surgery is sometimes unavoidable.

Removing your prostate and seminal vesicles will cause you to have dry orgasms. This means there will be no semen, which would prevent you from having children. You may want to look into sperm banking before the surgery if you're thinking of having children.

The recovery of erectile function is often frustratingly slow. It may take several months to 2 years to restore the erectile function you had before the prostatectomy. However, you may never regain the same erectile function you once had.

Treatment options for erectile dysfunction include pills (like Viagra and Cialis), injections of medication into the penis, vacuum constriction devices (penis pump), and surgical implants that produce an erection. You may need to try more than one treatment option to find out which can work for you.

Erectile dysfunction is also a common cause of psychological as well as relationship problems. It's a leading cause of depression in people with prostate cancer. Many individuals find it helpful to speak with a counselor or sex therapist after surgery.

Ask your doctor or someone else on your care team about therapy or counseling if you're having problems due to erectile dysfunction or symptoms of depression.

While it may be uncomfortable to talk about these problems, keep in mind that these side effects are common and help is readily available. You're not alone—emotional support is part of good cancer care.

Radiation therapy

Radiation therapy uses high-energy beams, like x-rays, to kill cancer cells and shrink tumors. Radiation therapy is given in regular doses over several to many days.

Radiation therapy has been shown to be as effective as surgery for early-stage prostate cancer. Decisions between the 2 options are generally made based on their potential side effects.

Radiation therapy is used in several ways to treat prostate cancer. It's used as primary therapy for prostate cancer, similar to surgery. It's also used after prostate surgery to kill any cancer cells that have been left behind.

Radiation therapy is also used to treat metastatic areas (where prostate cancer has spread to other parts of the body) to curb cancer growth or to relieve pain.

There are 2 main types of radiation treatment for prostate cancer: Radiation from outside the body (external beam radiation therapy) and radiation from inside the body (brachytherapy).

EBRT

External beam radiation therapy (EBRT) uses a large machine to deliver radiation from outside the body to a precise area inside the body. The radiation is focused directly on the cancer while trying to avoid healthy tissue.

EBRT requires careful planning. Before treatment, you may have tiny metal markers, each about the size of a grain of rice, implanted in your prostate.

These markers make sure the radiation beams are accurately aligned with your prostate in the same way for every treatment. This is done to improve the safety and effectiveness of the therapy.

You may also be given an injection of biodegradable gel between your prostate and rectum. The gel temporarily widens the area, which creates a space that helps protect the rectum from unwanted radiation during treatment.

Next, you may have a radiation simulation or mapping scan about 1 or 2 weeks before you begin therapy. This scan is used to design your personalized treatment plan. You'll lie on the treatment table and get into the best position for receiving the radiation. But you won't receive any actual radiation during the simulation. Sometimes a custom mold is made of your body to help you lie in the same position on the treatment table each day.

During the treatment itself, the machine may rotate around the table to deliver radiation from several different angles. You won't be able to see or feel the radiation when it's delivered.

External beam radiation therapy

External beam radiation therapy (EBRT) uses a machine that precisely aims radiation at cancer inside the body. The radiation beam focuses on the cancer while avoiding healthy tissue. This allows for safer delivery of higher doses of radiation to the cancer.

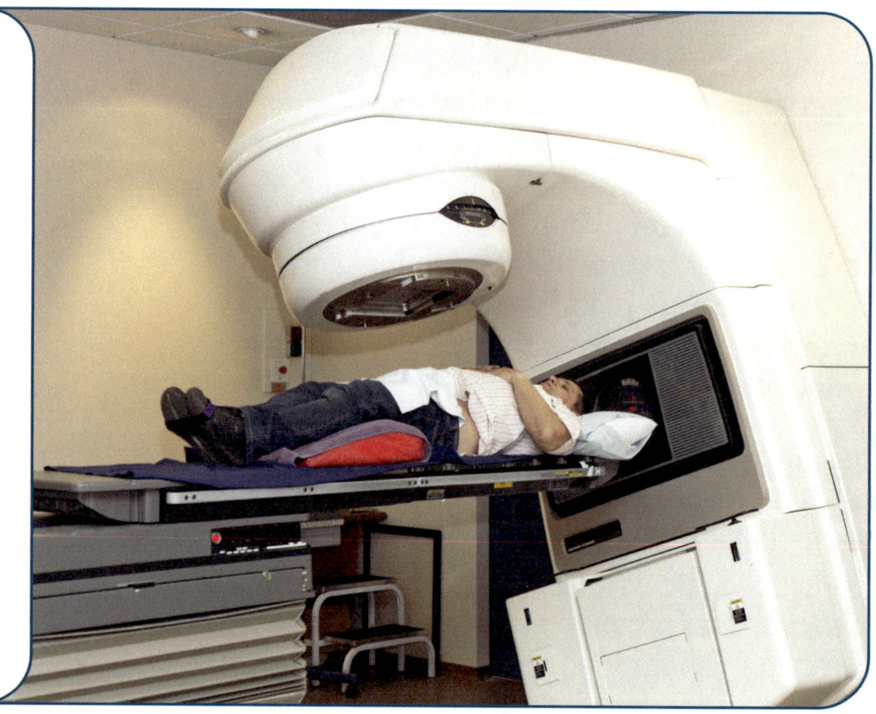

The total number of treatments varies from 5 to as many as 40. They're typically given in daily doses 5 days a week, Monday through Friday, over a period of weeks. A very precise, high-dose radiation treatment called stereotactic body radiation therapy (SBRT) is commonly given every other day for 5 treatments.

Proton beam therapy is a type of EBRT that uses protons instead of x-rays to deliver radiation to the cancer. Protons are tiny, electrically charged particles smaller than an atom. Researchers have found that proton beam therapy has the same effect on prostate cancer and the same risk for side effects as EBRT.

Brachytherapy

Brachytherapy is an internal form of radiation therapy. You might hear it called brachy (pronounced "BRAY-key") for short. In this treatment, radiation is delivered inside the body by placing a radioactive object into or next to the tumor. Brachytherapy is a minimally invasive procedure and is often done under general anesthesia like a surgical procedure.

Brachytherapy may be used alone or combined with EBRT, hormone therapy, or both. Patients with high-risk cancers aren't usually considered for brachytherapy alone.

High dose-rate brachytherapy involves a procedure where 10 to 20 very narrow tubes are inserted through the perineum (the skin between the anus and scrotum) and into your prostate. Thin wires with radioactive tips slide through the tubes and are held within the prostate for several minutes.

Brachytherapy radiation

Low dose-rate brachytherapy uses tiny radioactive metal "seeds" that are implanted into your prostate. Each seed is about the size of a grain of rice. They'll stay in your prostate permanently and provide a low dose of radiation continuously for several months.

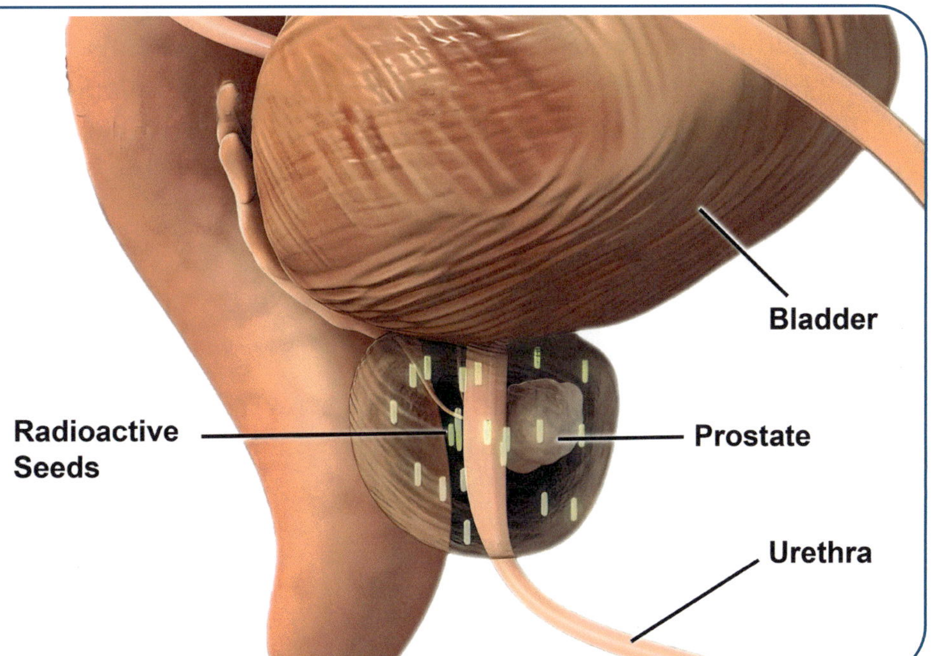

During this time, the tips deliver a high dose of radiation to the prostate. The wires are then retracted and the needles are removed, leaving no radioactive material behind.

Low dose-rate brachytherapy is delivered by as many as 50 tiny metal "seeds" that are permanently implanted in your prostate. The seeds gradually release a continuous low dose of radiation over months.

Side effects of radiation therapy

Common side effects of radiation therapy are urinary and bowel problems, erectile dysfunction, and fatigue.

Urinary and bowel problems – Urinary problems include having to go more often, having to go suddenly, a burning sensation when you go and, rarely, blood in the urine. Bowel problems are much less common with modern forms of radiation but can include diarrhea, pooping frequently, being unable to hold poop in and, rarely, bleeding from the rectum.

Urinary and bowel problems usually lessen or go away after several weeks for most people, but may last longer for others.

Erectile dysfunction – Radiation therapy is less likely than surgery to cause erectile dysfunction. But radiation can damage the vessels and nerves that control erections.

Erectile dysfunction doesn't happen right away after radiation. It usually occurs gradually, starting and then worsening between 1 to 3 years after radiation treatment. Having hormone therapy in addition to radiation therapy can make this side effect more likely. (For more information, see "Erectile dysfunction" on page 39.)

Medications are often (but not always) effective for erectile dysfunction after radiation therapy.

Fatigue – Feeling tired for a few weeks to months after radiation therapy is also common. Regular physical activity and exercise can help relieve mild fatigue.

Other cancer – It's rare, but radiation therapy slightly increases the risk for developing another cancer in the pelvis, such as bladder or rectal cancer.

Hormone therapy

Hormone therapy is a treatment that adds, blocks, or removes hormones. A hormone is a natural chemical made by a gland in the body. Its job is to activate cells or organs.

Male hormones are called androgens. The main androgen is testosterone. Most of the testosterone in the body is made by the testicles. Testosterone helps produce sperm, among other functions.

But testosterone also helps prostate cancer grow. A type of hormone therapy called androgen deprivation therapy (ADT) can stop your body from making testosterone or block cancer cells from using testosterone. This can shrink the tumor or slow tumor growth for a while.

Hormone therapies for prostate cancer

Hormone therapies for prostate cancer include luteinizing hormone-releasing hormone (LHRH) agonists and LHRH antagonists, both of which cause the testicles to stop making testosterone.

Most LHRH agonists and LHRH antagonists are injections. They may be given monthly or 2, 3, or 4 times a year. Relugolix (Orgovyx) is an LHRH antagonist that comes as a tablet taken once a day.

Other hormone therapies include anti-androgens and androgen synthesis inhibitors. Anti-androgens block prostate cancer cells from using androgens to grow. Androgen synthesis inhibitors prevent the glands—and the cancer itself—from making androgen. These therapies are available as pills and taken 1 to 3 times a day, depending on the medication. See **Guide 5**.

Hormone therapy isn't recommended to be used by itself for the treatment of early-stage prostate cancer. When hormone therapy is used (generally for higher risk prostate cancer), it's usually given with radiation therapy, which increases radiation's effectiveness. Hormone therapy is often started before radiation therapy begins and is typically continued during and after radiation therapy.

You might hear the term **castration** used when describing prostate cancer or its treatment. This term describes a drastic reduction of testosterone. Castration can be done with hormone-lowering medication or by surgical removal of one or both testicles (orchiectomy).

Although orchiectomy is a surgical procedure, it's still considered hormone therapy because it removes the primary source of testosterone: the testicles. While hormone drug therapy can be reversed when the medication is stopped,

Guide 5
Hormone therapy drugs for early-stage prostate cancer

LHRH agonists	Goserelin (Zoladex), leuprolide (Lupron Depot, Eligard), triptorelin (Trelstar)
LHRH antagonists	Degarelix (Firmagon), relugolix (Orgovyx)
Anti-androgens	Bicalutamide (Casodex), flutamide (Eulexin), nilutamide (Nilandron)
Androgen synthesis inhibitors	**Very high-risk cancer only:** Abiraterone (Zytiga)

orchiectomy is permanent and can't be reversed.

Surgical removal of the testicles is much less common today because hormone drug therapy is often just as effective at blocking testosterone. Still, some individuals (often those with metastatic prostate cancer) prefer this one-time procedure over daily medications or periodic injections.

Side effects of hormone therapy

Hormone therapy can have significant side effects. Many factors affect your risk for side effects, including your age, your health before treatment, how long or often you have treatment, and other things.

In general, the longer you're on hormone therapy, the greater your risk for side effects.

Hot flashes are one of the most common side effects of hormone therapy. A hot flash is a sudden feeling of warmth that may turn your face red and cause you to sweat.

Other side effects include tiredness (fatigue), mood changes, weight gain, changes in penis length and testicle size, tenderness and growth of your breasts, and loss of muscle mass.

Sexual side effects – The sexual side effects of hormone therapy are a significant cause of stress. Hormone therapy may lower your desire for sex, cause erectile dysfunction, and reduce the size of the penis and testicles.

Erectile dysfunction medicines (such as Viagra and Cialis) aren't usually effective for people on hormone therapy. But there are some injected medicines that may be helpful. These drugs don't restore the loss of sexual desire caused by lower androgen levels, though.

Loss of sex drive, erectile dysfunction, and other sexual side effects usually go away after you stop hormone therapy. But it may take a

NCCN experts are concerned about overtreatment of early-stage prostate cancer. For many people, observation or active surveillance are better options.

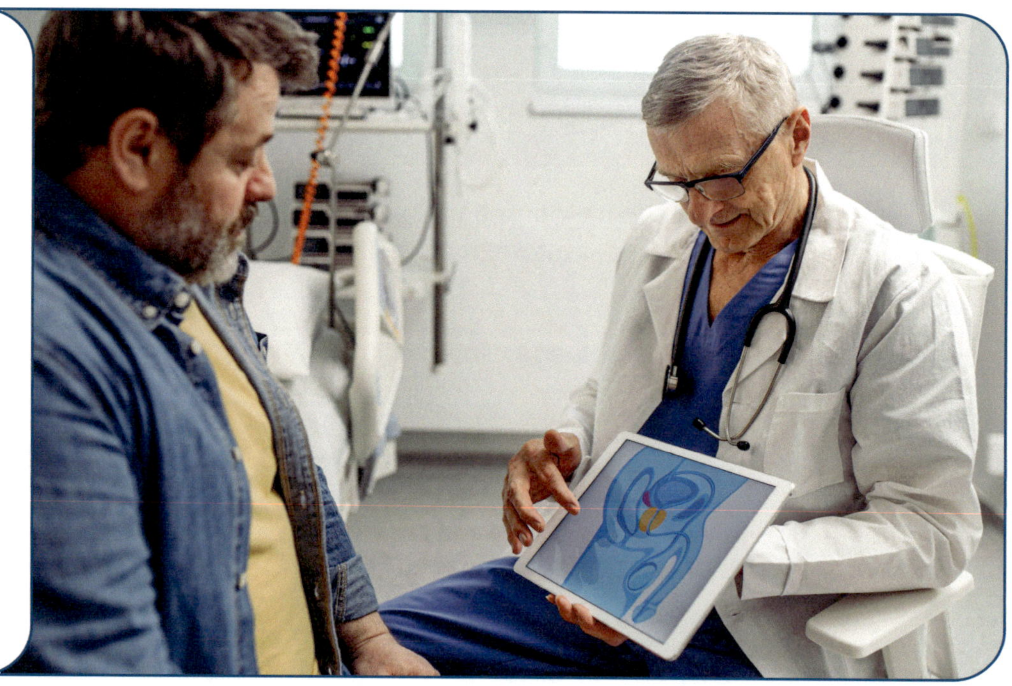

year or more to regain your testosterone level and libido (sex drive). Many patients never fully regain the same levels of testosterone and libido that they had before hormone therapy. Some never regain the full ability to have an erection.

In the meantime, consider talking to your partner and/or a therapist to help you deal with any challenges you're having. You're not alone—emotional support is an important part of cancer care.

Bone thinning and fractures – Thinning and weakening of your bones (osteoporosis) and bone fractures can also happen. When you start ADT, you'll have a test to measure your bone density. If your bone density is low, your care team can recommend medications to strengthen your bones. Taking daily calcium and vitamin D can also help keep your bones strong while you're on ADT.

Diabetes and heart disease – Hormone therapy also increases the risk for diabetes and cardiovascular disease. If you already have either of these conditions, hormone therapy can make them worse. Hormone therapy may also increase the risk for death from heart issues. Be sure to talk to your care team about your personal risk.

Testosterone flare – LHRH agonists can cause a surge in testosterone for a few weeks before it drops to an undetectable level. This increase is called a testosterone flare. A testosterone flare can cause bone pain and urinary problems. These symptoms will go away after the first few weeks of hormone therapy. But you may be given an anti-androgen medicine to prevent testosterone flare until then.

☑ **TIP**

Regular exercise can lessen the symptoms and side effects of hormone therapy, including:

- Weight gain
- Fatigue
- Loss of bone and muscle mass

Physical activity can also improve your general health and make you feel better. Ask your care team to recommend an exercise program for you.

Talk to your care team about how to manage the side effects of hormone therapy. They have ways to lessen or soothe most of these difficulties. Bones can be strengthened with medicine as well as with physical activity.

Exercise and eating a healthy diet can also help with fatigue, mood, and maintaining a healthy weight.

Clinical trials

Another way to receive treatment for prostate cancer may be through a clinical trial.

A clinical trial is a type of medical research study. After being developed and tested in a lab, potential new ways of fighting cancer need to be studied in people.

If found to be safe and effective in a clinical trial, a drug, device, or treatment approach may be approved by the U.S. FDA.

Everyone with cancer should carefully consider all of the treatment options available for their cancer type, including standard treatments and clinical trials. Talk to your doctor about whether a clinical trial may make sense for you.

Phases

Most cancer clinical trials focus on treatment and are done in phases.

- **Phase 1** trials study the safety and side effects of an investigational drug or treatment approach.
- **Phase 2** trials study how well the drug or approach works against a specific type of cancer.
- **Phase 3** trials test the drug or approach against a standard treatment. If the results are good, it may be approved by the FDA.
- **Phase 4** trials study the safety and benefit of an FDA-approved treatment.

Who can enroll?

It depends on the clinical trial's rules, called eligibility criteria. The rules may be about age, cancer type and stage, treatment history, or general health. They ensure that participants are alike in specific ways and that the trial is as safe as possible for the participants.

Everyone with cancer can ask for and should be given information about clinical trials.

Knowing all of your options means not missing out on clinical trial opportunities for promising new treatments.

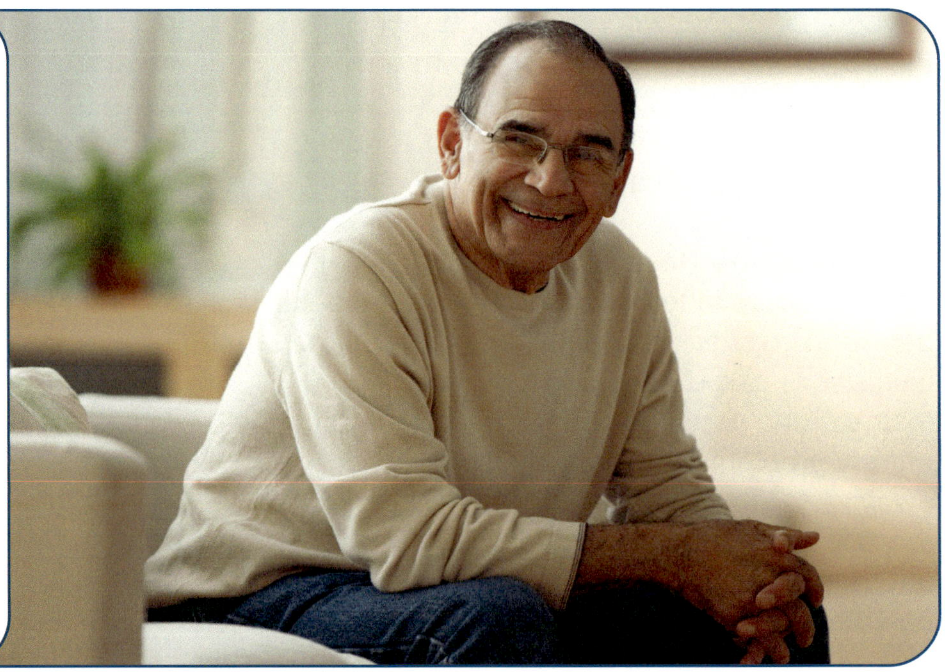

> **Without clinical trials, our treatment wouldn't change. It would always remain the same. Some people refer to clinical trials as receiving tomorrow's best treatment today."**

Informed consent

Clinical trials are managed by a research team. This group of experts will review the study with you in detail, including its purpose and the risks and benefits of joining.

All of this information is also provided in an informed consent form. Read the form carefully and ask questions before signing it. Take time to discuss it with people you trust.

Keep in mind that you can leave and seek treatment outside of the clinical trial at any time.

Will I get a placebo?

Placebos (inactive versions of real medicines) are almost never used alone in cancer clinical trials. It is common to receive either a placebo with a standard treatment, or a new drug with a standard treatment.

You will be informed, verbally and in writing, if a placebo is part of a clinical trial before you enroll.

Finding a clinical trial

In the United States

NCCN Cancer Centers
NCCN.org/cancercenters

The National Cancer Institute (NCI)
cancer.gov/about-cancer/treatment/clinical-trials/search

Worldwide

The U.S. National Library of Medicine (NLM)
clinicaltrials.gov

Need help finding a clinical trial?

NCI's Cancer Information Service (CIS)
1.800.4.CANCER (1.800.422.6237)
cancer.gov/contact

Are clinical trials free?

There is no fee to enroll in a clinical trial. The study sponsor pays for research-related costs, including the study drug. But you may need to pay for other services, like transportation or childcare, due to extra appointments. During the trial, you will continue to receive standard cancer care. This care is often covered by insurance.

Supportive care

Supportive care is an important part of cancer care. The goal is to improve your quality of life during and after cancer treatment. Supportive care is for everyone with cancer and their families, not just for those at the end of life. It's also known as palliative care.

Supportive care includes a wide range of services. Supportive care prevents or manages the symptoms of cancer and the side effects of cancer treatment, like pain and cancer-related fatigue. It also addresses the mental, social, emotional, and spiritual concerns faced by people with cancer.

Supportive care provides help with additional needs, such as:

- Making treatment decisions
- Coordinating your care
- Paying for care
- Planning for advance care and end of life

People who start supportive care when they begin treatment tend to have improved outcomes and better quality of life.

Supportive care involves the whole person, not just their cancer. If you're having a problem that's interfering with your treatment or affecting your quality of life, ask what supportive care resources may be available to help you.

Read more about the types of support you may receive in the *NCCN Guidelines for Patients: Palliative Care*, available at NCCN.org/patientguidelines and on the NCCN Patient Guides for Cancer app.

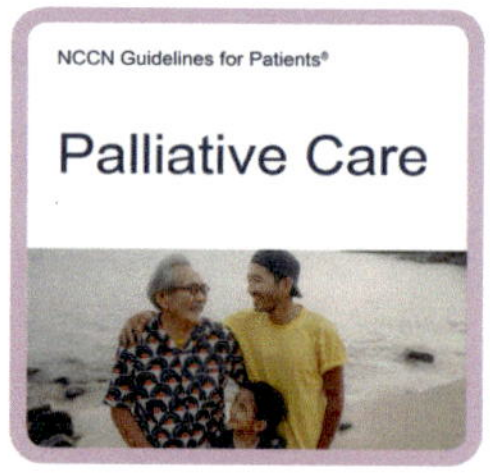

Support groups

Many people diagnosed with cancer find support groups to be helpful. A support group provides the opportunity to talk with others who are going through, or have been through, similar experiences.

Support groups often include people at different stages of treatment. Some people may be newly diagnosed, while others may be finished with treatment.

If your hospital or community doesn't have support groups for people with prostate cancer, check out the websites listed on pages 71–72 of this guide.

Your treatment goals

Everyone's cancer and life situation are different. Here's a step-by-step self-assessment to help you think about what matters most to you, so you can talk with your doctor and care team about your goals for treatment.

Step 1: Understanding shared decision-making

Your doctor is the expert on prostate cancer and its treatments. You are the expert on **you**—your body, values, and life priorities. Working together with your doctors and care team helps create a plan that fits both your medical needs and your personal goals. This is called shared decision-making.

Step 2: What matters most to you?

Below are examples of common treatment goals. Check (✓) any that are important to you or add your own in the blank spaces.

Step 3: Questions to ask your care team

Use the questions at the end of each chapter of this guide to begin conversations with your doctors and care team.

Step 4: Review and revisit your goals

Your goals may change over time as your treatment and life circumstances evolve. Revisit this self-assessment regularly and share updates with your care team.

Your health and treatment goals

- ☐ Live as long and as well as possible
- ☐ Prevent or control symptoms such as pain, fatigue, and urinary difficulties
- ☐ Prevent or delay further growth or spread of the cancer
- ☐ Keep treatment side effects manageable

Your quality of life goals

- ☐ Maintain my daily activities
- ☐ Retain the ability to have an erection
- ☐ Avoid or minimalize the loss of urinary control
- ☐ Manage the financial cost of treatment
- ☐ Keep my independence and mobility
- ☐ Feel informed and involved in every treatment decision
- ☐ Spend quality time with my family and friends

Add your other personal goals or concerns

- ☐ ______________________________
- ☐ ______________________________
- ☐ ______________________________

Key points

- Active surveillance is the preferred strategy for most people who have lower-risk prostate cancer and a longer life expectancy.
- Radical prostatectomy is prostate surgery that removes the whole prostate, the surrounding tissue, the seminal vesicles, and sometimes the nearby lymph nodes in the pelvis.
- Radiation therapy precisely targets prostate cancer to kill cancer cells and stop new cancer cells from being made.
- Hormone therapy treats prostate cancer by stopping testosterone from being made or by blocking cancer cells from using testosterone.
- Castration describes a drastic reduction of testosterone. This is most often done with drugs.
- Supportive care is important at any stage of cancer, not just at the end of life.

Questions to ask

- Do I have a choice of when to begin treatment?
- How long do I have to decide what to do?
- Does any option offer a cure or long-term cancer control?
- Which side effects are most common and how long do they usually last?
- What supportive care and services are available to me and my caregivers?

"I realized there were only a few variables within my control: Sleep, diet, exercise, spending time with family and friends, and a positive mental attitude. I focused on the things I could personally affect and put all of the what-ifs out of my mind."

6

Initial treatment for your risk group

You've had a lot of tests to determine your risk group. Now, you and your care team will use your risk assessment to decide your initial treatment options.

Has your doctor or care team told you which risk group you're in? If you know your risk group, look for it in the following pages to learn about your initial therapy options.

Low risk

The low-risk group includes patients who have all of the following traits:

- Tumor stage T1 to T2a
- Grade Group 1
- Prostate-specific antigen (PSA) less than 10 ng/mL

NCCN experts are concerned about overtreatment of early-stage prostate cancer. One result of overtreatment is that the treatment might cause more problems than the disease itself. For many patients, especially those with low-risk prostate cancer, active surveillance or observation can be better options than direct treatment.

Management options are based on life expectancy estimates. The initial management options for low-risk prostate cancer are described next and shown in **Guide 6**.

Life expectancy: 10 years or more

If you have low-risk prostate cancer and your estimated life expectancy is 10 years or more, you're likely to receive active surveillance.

Active surveillance
Active surveillance means that your care team will watch your condition closely and will be ready to start treatment if needed.

Guide 6
Low-risk group: Initial management options

Life expectancy estimate	Initial therapy	Followed by
10 years or more	Active surveillance (preferred)	
	Radiation therapy	Tests for PSA recurrence
	Prostate surgery*	Tests for PSA persistence and recurrence
Less than 10 years	Observation	

**See Guide 8 for adverse features.*

Active surveillance is the preferred option if you have slow-growing prostate cancer and a longer life expectancy.

Tests during active surveillance include PSA, digital rectal exam, MRI scan, and biopsies. These tests are done on a regular basis so that treatment can be started when and if needed. See **Guide 7**.

To see if you're a good candidate for active surveillance, you may need a confirmatory MRI scan (if you haven't had an MRI already). The confirmatory MRI can be done with or without a confirmatory prostate biopsy and/or biomarker testing.

All patients should have a confirmatory prostate biopsy 1 to 2 years after their initial biopsy to see if any changes have happened over time.

Radiation therapy

If you're likely to live more than 10 years, you may decide you want treatment now instead of active surveillance. Low-risk cancers can be treated with radiation therapy, either external beam radiation therapy (EBRT) or brachytherapy.

> **It's important to understand what you're going through. If your doctor says something you don't understand, don't just nod like you do. Let them know "I don't understand what that means" or "I don't fully understand what you just said. Can you please explain it in simpler terms?"**

Guide 7
Tests during active surveillance

Test	Frequency
PSA test	Once or twice a year, or as needed
Digital rectal exam	Once a year, or as needed
MRI scan	Every 1 to 2 years, or as needed
Prostate biopsy	Every 1 to 3 years, or as needed

Prostate surgery

Prostate surgery (radical prostatectomy) removes the whole prostate. It's not a common treatment option for people with low-risk prostate cancer.

After the prostate is removed, the pathologist will look for signs of disease called adverse (or high-risk) features. See **Guide 8**. Having any adverse features suggests that not all of the cancer was removed during surgery.

Even if you have any adverse features, the preferred strategy for low-risk prostate cancer is monitoring. Monitoring involves periodic PSA tests and possibly digital rectal exams. If your PSA level rises during monitoring, you'll have further tests to see if the cancer has returned.

If test results don't show adverse features, then you'll be monitored for cancer recurrence.

Life expectancy: Less than 10 years

If you have low-risk prostate cancer and your life expectancy is less than 10 years, observation is often recommended.

Observation

Observation is for people whose prostate cancer isn't causing any symptoms and who have other, more serious health conditions.

Observation involves occasional PSA tests and watching for symptoms, which can be treated with palliative care.

Guide 8
Adverse features that may be found after prostate surgery

If tests show any of these high-risk features after prostate surgery, you may need additional therapy:	• Cancer in the edge of the tissue removed in prostate surgery (surgical margin) • Cancer outside the layer surrounding the prostate • Cancer in the seminal vesicle(s)

About intermediate-risk groups

Intermediate-risk prostate cancer hasn't grown outside of the prostate itself. It doesn't have high-risk or very high-risk features, but it does have **1 or more** of the following intermediate risk factors:

- Tumor stage T2b or T2c
- Grade Group 2 or 3
- PSA 10 to 20 ng/mL

The intermediate-risk group is further divided into **favorable** and **unfavorable** subgroups.

Treatment is based on whether your prostate cancer has favorable intermediate risk or unfavorable intermediate risk.

Favorable intermediate risk

People who have only 1 of the following traits have favorable intermediate risk:

- Tumor stage T2b or T2c
- Grade Group 2
- PSA 10 to 20 ng/mL

In addition to having 1 of these traits, another indication of favorable intermediate risk is that fewer than half of the cores removed during your biopsy show cancer.

Treatment options for people with favorable intermediate-risk cancer are shown in **Guide 9**. Treatment options are based on life expectancy estimates.

Guide 9
Favorable intermediate-risk group: Initial therapy options

Life expectancy estimate	Initial therapy	Followed by
10 years or more	Active surveillance	
	Radiation therapy	Tests for PSA recurrence
	Prostate surgery*	Tests for PSA persistence and recurrence
5 to 10 years	Observation (preferred)	
	Radiation therapy	Tests for PSA recurrence

**See Guide 8 for adverse features.*

Life expectancy: 10 years or more

If you have favorable intermediate-risk prostate cancer and your estimated life expectancy is 10 years or more, your initial treatment options include active surveillance, radiation therapy, or perhaps prostate surgery.

Active surveillance

Active surveillance consists of testing on a regular basis so that treatment can be started when needed.

To see if you're a good candidate for active surveillance, you'll need a confirmatory MRI scan (if you haven't had an MRI already) and a confirmatory prostate biopsy with or without biomarker testing. Confirmatory testing is a way to check that your prostate cancer isn't worse than it appears.

People in the favorable intermediate-risk group who are particularly good candidates for active surveillance have a low percentage of Gleason pattern 4 cancer, low volume disease (in which fewer biopsy core samples contain cancer), low PSA density, and/or low genomic risk.

Active surveillance is **not** recommended for people in the favorable intermediate risk group whose cancer cells, when looked at under a microscope, indicate a higher risk for aggressive or recurrent cancer. Radical prostatectomy or radiation therapy are more effective options in these cases.

After treatment for favorable intermediate-risk prostate cancer, your PSA level will be watched closely for any changes. See **Guide 9**.

Radiation therapy

Radiation therapy is a treatment option for some individuals with favorable intermediate-risk prostate cancer. Whether it's an option for you may depend on several factors, including the size of the tumor or the results of a specialized risk test. Radiation treatments include either EBRT or brachytherapy.

Prostate surgery

If you're expected to live an estimated 10 years or more, surgery to remove your prostate (radical prostatectomy) may be an option.

Occasionally, the pelvic lymph nodes may also be removed in individuals with favorable intermediate-risk prostate cancer. (Your doctor can estimate the risk for cancer in these lymph nodes using a nomogram.) A surgical procedure called a pelvic lymph node dissection is performed to remove the nodes and check them for cancer.

If any adverse features are found in your prostate (see **Guide 8**), the preferred option is to be monitored rather than have additional treatment right away. Additional treatment, if needed, is typically radiation with or without hormone therapy.

After your treatment, your team will monitor you for any sign of the cancer coming back (recurrence). Monitoring involves periodic PSA tests and possibly digital rectal exams. If your PSA level rises during monitoring, you'll have further tests to see if the cancer has returned.

Life expectancy: Between 5 and 10 years

If you have favorable intermediate-risk prostate cancer and your estimated life expectancy is between 5 and 10 years, options include observation or perhaps radiation therapy.

Observation
Observation is the preferred option for people in this situation. Observation involves occasional PSA tests and watching for symptoms, which can be treated with palliative care.

Radiation therapy
Radiation therapy is a treatment option for some people whose favorable intermediate-risk cancer may grow or develop symptoms in their lifetime. Radiation treatments include either EBRT or brachytherapy.

Unfavorable intermediate risk

People in the unfavorable intermediate-risk subgroup have Grade Group 3 prostate cancer **or** cancer in more than half of their biopsy core samples. They also have 1 or 2 of the following traits:

- Tumor stage T2b or T2c
- PSA 10 to 20 ng/mL

Treatment options for unfavorable intermediate-risk prostate cancer are shown in **Guide 10**. Treatment options are based on life expectancy.

Guide 10
Unfavorable intermediate-risk group: Initial therapy options

Life expectancy estimate	Initial therapy	Followed by
10 years or more	Prostate surgery with or without pelvic lymph node removal*	Tests for PSA persistence and recurrence
	Radiation therapy and ADT	Tests for PSA recurrence
5 to 10 years	Observation	
	Radiation therapy and ADT	Tests for PSA recurrence

**See Guide 8 for adverse features.*

Life expectancy: 10 years or more

If you have unfavorable intermediate-risk prostate cancer and your estimated life expectancy is 10 years or more, your initial treatment options include radical prostatectomy or radiation with hormone therapy.

Prostate surgery

Surgically removing the prostate (radical prostatectomy) is a recommended option for people in this risk group.

Your pelvic lymph nodes may also be removed if there's a small risk for the cancer to spread to them. (Your doctor will determine this risk using a nomogram.) A surgical procedure called a pelvic lymph node dissection is performed to remove the nodes and check them for cancer.

If you have any adverse features (see **Guide 8**), the preferred option is to be monitored rather than have additional treatment.

If test results don't find high-risk features after prostate surgery, then your treatment team will monitor you for any sign of the cancer coming back (recurrence). Monitoring involves periodic PSA tests and possibly digital rectal exams. If your PSA level rises during monitoring, you'll have further tests to see if the cancer has returned.

Radiation and hormone therapy

Radiation therapy with hormone therapy is also an initial treatment option for people with unfavorable intermediate-risk cancer and life expectancy of 10 years or more.

Radiation therapy options include EBRT or brachytherapy. The type of radiation therapy you receive will depend on several factors including the extent of the cancer.

Hormone therapy involves 4 to 6 months of androgen deprivation therapy (ADT), preferably done during and after radiation therapy.

Radiation therapy combined with long-term hormone therapy can be an effective initial treatment for people at high risk or very high risk.

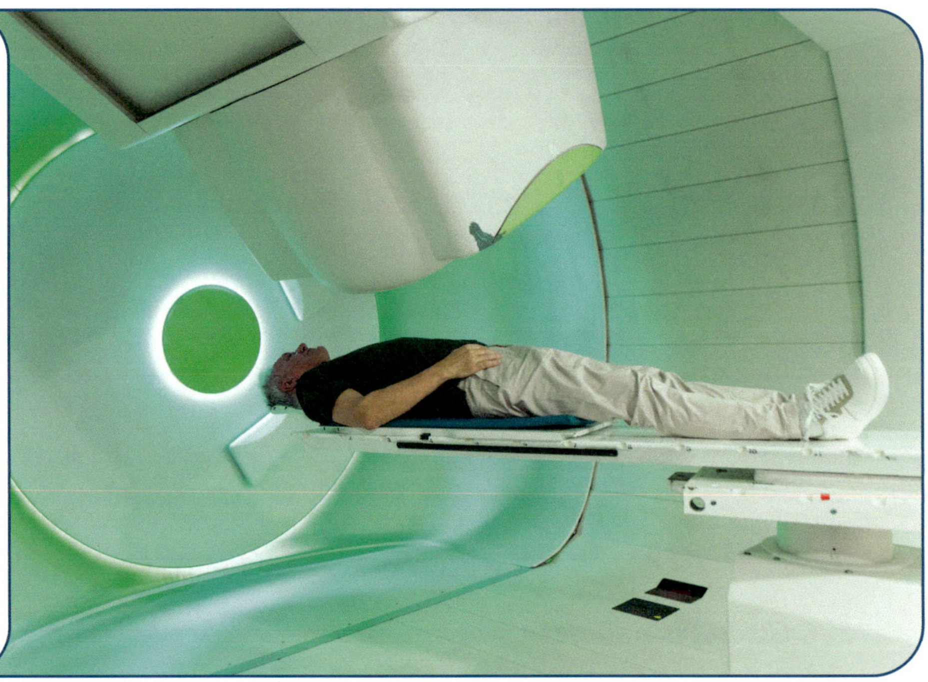

Life expectancy: Between 5 and 10 years

If you have unfavorable intermediate-risk prostate cancer and your estimated life expectancy is 5 to 10 years, your options include observation or radiation plus hormone therapy.

Observation
Because the cancer may progress too slowly to cause problems within 5 to 10 years, active surveillance is not recommended for people in this risk group. Observation is the recommended option instead.

Observation involves occasional PSA tests and watching for symptoms, which can be treated with palliative care.

Radiation and hormone therapy
Radiation therapy plus hormone therapy (ADT) is also an option for individuals in the unfavorable intermediate-risk group with an estimated life expectancy between 5 and 10 years.

Radiation treatment involves EBRT or brachytherapy, plus 4 to 6 months of hormone therapy. You should receive hormone therapy preferably during and after radiation therapy, rather than before it.

High risk or very high risk

The **high-risk** group includes people whose cancer has at least 1 of the following characteristics:

- Tumor stage T3 to T4
- Grade Group 4 or 5
- PSA more than 20 ng/mL

The **very high-risk** group includes those whose cancer has at least 2 of these characteristics:

- Tumor stage T3 to T4
- Grade Group 4 or 5
- PSA more than 40 ng/mL

Treatment is more aggressive for high-risk and very high-risk prostate cancer. Treatment options are based on life expectancy and whether or not you have symptoms. See **Guide 11**.

Life expectancy: More than 5 years or you have symptoms

If your estimated life expectancy is more than 5 years or you have symptoms, there are several options for initial therapy:

Radiation and hormone therapy
Radiation therapy combined with long-term hormone therapy can be an effective initial treatment for high-risk or very high-risk prostate cancer.

For this treatment, hormone therapy is given before, during, and after EBRT for 18 months to 3 years.

Another radiation therapy option, if available, is EBRT combined with brachytherapy and long-term hormone therapy (1 to 3 years).

Combining EBRT and brachytherapy allows for more careful control of the radiation dose. When hormone therapy is added to this combination, patient outcomes tend to improve.

A shorter course of hormone therapy (1 year) is sometimes given to certain individuals receiving this treatment combination.

There's also a treatment option only for certain individuals with very high-risk prostate cancer: Abiraterone (Zytiga) can be combined with radiation therapy and 2 years of hormone therapy.

Prostate surgery

For individuals estimated to live more than 5 years, a radical prostatectomy is an option for those in the high-risk group and certain individuals in the very high-risk group. Your age and overall health will be factors in deciding if this is a good option for you.

Guide 11
High-risk and very high-risk groups: Initial therapy options

Life expectancy estimate	Initial therapy	Followed by
More than 5 years or you have symptoms	Radiation therapy and ADT	Tests for PSA recurrence
	Very high-risk cancer only: Radiation therapy, ADT, and Abiraterone (Zytiga)	Tests for PSA recurrence
	Prostate surgery*	Tests for PSA persistence and recurrence
5 years or less and you have no symptoms	Observation	
	Radiation therapy and ADT	Tests for PSA recurrence
	Radiation therapy	Tests for PSA recurrence

**See Guide 8 for adverse features.*

After surgery, the removed prostate tissue will be tested. You might need to have additional treatment if cancer has spread to the lymph nodes or if adverse (high-risk) features are found (see **Guide 8**).

- **No adverse features found** – If test results find no adverse features in the prostate tissue, no additional treatment is needed. Your cancer will be monitored. Monitoring involves periodic PSA tests and possibly digital rectal exams. If your PSA level begins to rise during monitoring, you may need treatment for PSA recurrence.
- **Adverse features found** – If test results find adverse features but no cancer in the lymph nodes after surgery, the preferred option is to be monitored for cancer recurrence. Additional treatment, typically EBRT and perhaps hormone therapy, is also an option.
- **Cancer found in lymph nodes** – If your prostate surgery shows that cancer has spread to your lymph nodes but you have no other adverse features, then additional treatment using radiation with or without hormone therapy may be your next option. Monitoring is also a reasonable choice if your PSA level is undetectable. However, if your PSA level begins to rise during monitoring, you may need treatment for PSA recurrence.

Additional treatment and PSA recurrence are discussed in *Chapter 7: PSA persistence and recurrence*.

Supportive care

In addition to these treatments, you may also receive supportive care (palliative care).

Supportive care is for relieving the symptoms caused by cancer and the side effects caused by cancer treatment.

Life expectancy: 5 years or less and no symptoms

If you have high-risk or very high-risk cancer and are expected to live an estimated 5 years or less, you should undergo bone imaging to see if the cancer has spread to any bones. You might also have imaging of your abdomen and pelvis to look for cancer in the lymph nodes and areas near the prostate. Finding cancer in these areas will affect what treatment you receive. See **Guide 11**.

But if the cancer **has not** spread to any bones, lymph nodes, or organs, then 3 options are available:

Observation

For people with higher-risk cancer and shorter life expectancy, the best treatment may be no treatment. Observation mainly involves occasional PSA tests and watching for symptoms, which can be treated with palliative care.

Radiation and hormone therapy

Radiation therapy combined with long-term hormone therapy can be an effective primary treatment for high-risk or very high-risk cancer. Hormone therapy is given before, during, and after EBRT for 18 months to 3 years.

Radiation therapy

EBRT by itself is a treatment option for certain people with high-risk or very high-risk prostate cancer. Brachytherapy by itself isn't an option, but it may be added to EBRT for a boost of radiation therapy in high-risk or very high-risk prostate cancer.

Supportive care
In addition to these treatments, you may also receive supportive care (palliative care). Supportive care is for relieving the symptoms caused by cancer and the side effects caused by cancer treatment.

Tests after treatment

After your initial treatment, you'll be monitored for any increase in PSA or cancer recurrence. Monitoring involves these follow-up tests:

- PSA test every 6 to 12 months for 5 years, then once a year after that
- Possibly a digital rectal exam if your doctor suspects cancer recurrence

PSA testing may be done more often in people with high-risk or very high-risk prostate cancer.

If your PSA level (or digital rectal exam, if performed) indicates the cancer has returned, then you might need imaging, biopsy, or additional (or different) treatment. See *Chapter 7: PSA persistence and recurrence*.

Key points

- Anyone receiving active surveillance should have a confirmatory prostate biopsy 1 to 2 years after their initial biopsy.
- If there's a risk that cancer has spread or will spread to lymph nodes in the pelvis, you can have a procedure to remove the lymph nodes and check them for cancer.
- If you have any adverse features after a radical prostatectomy, you'll likely be monitored rather than have additional treatment.
- If your PSA level begins to rise after treatment, you may need additional treatment for PSA recurrence. If your PSA level doesn't lower enough after treatment, you may need additional treatment for PSA persistence.

Questions to ask

- How long will my treatment last?
- Will my insurance cover the treatment you're recommending?
- Are you suggesting options other than what NCCN recommends? If yes, why?
- How will you know if the treatment is working?
- What are the chances of the cancer worsening or returning?

7

PSA persistence and recurrence

Even after treatment with prostate surgery or radiation therapy, your prostate-specific antigen (PSA) level may not go down low enough. Or your PSA level may drop but, at some point, begin to rise again. These are usually signs that you'll need further treatment.

If you've had a radical prostatectomy, all the cells that make prostate-specific antigen (PSA) should have been removed by surgery. So your PSA level should become undetectable. If you had radiation therapy, your PSA level should fall steadily and remain at a low level.

But in about 1 in 3 people treated for localized prostate cancer (cancer that's only in the prostate), their PSA level either doesn't drop low enough (called PSA persistence) or it drops to near zero but eventually starts to rise again (called PSA recurrence).

PSA is considered persistent if it hasn't dropped low enough by the time you have your first PSA test after surgery.

PSA recurrence may not develop for several years after initial treatment.

PSA persistence and PSA recurrence may be signs that the cancer hasn't fully gone away or that it has come back in another part of the body. For these reasons, treatment for PSA persistence and PSA recurrence often includes both local and whole-body therapies. The local therapy is often radiation, while whole-body therapy involves hormone treatment.

Rising PSA isn't necessarily a cause for panic. There's usually time to decide on the right treatment. Sometimes no therapy is needed, and you can continue to be monitored.

If life expectancy is 5 years or less

Note that the treatment options listed in this chapter are for people with an estimated life expectancy of more than 5 years.

For individuals with an estimated life expectancy of 5 years or less, observation and supportive care (palliative care) may be more reasonable options than undergoing treatment and dealing with the side effects.

Testing for persistence or recurrence

Before deciding on any treatment, you'll have more tests to find out how aggressive the cancer is.

The first thing your care team will do is re-evaluate your risk. Many factors, not just your PSA level, are taken into consideration to figure out your current level of risk.

These factors commonly include:

- Your age
- Your overall health
- Which initial therapy you had and how long ago you had it
- If you have cancer in your lymph nodes or any other adverse factors
- How fast your PSA is rising

If necessary, additional testing may include another biopsy and whole-body imaging.

If tests find a rise in PSA or another sign of cancer, then you'll have a discussion with your care team about the risks and benefits of your possible treatment options.

Treatment for persistence or recurrence

If your life expectancy is estimated to be more than 5 years, treatment for persistence or recurrence is primarily based on whether your initial treatment was radical prostatectomy or radiation therapy. See **Guide 12**.

Guide 12
Treatments for PSA persistence or PSA recurrence: Life expectancy estimate is more than 5 years

Initial therapy	Test results	Management options for persistence or recurrence
Radical prostatectomy	Raised PSA, but no other signs of cancer found	• Radiation therapy (preferred) with or without androgen deprivation therapy (ADT) • Monitoring
	Cancer found in pelvic lymph nodes	• Radiation and ADT • Radiation and hormone therapy + abiraterone
	Cancer has spread to another area of the body (metastasized)	• Advanced treatment required
Radiation therapy	Raised PSA or abnormal digital rectal exam, but no other signs of cancer found or Cancer found only in the prostate or Cancer found in pelvic lymph nodes	• Monitoring • ADT • Radical prostatectomy and removal of pelvic lymph nodes with or without ADT • Cryotherapy with or without ADT • High-intensity focused ultrasound with or without ADT • Re-irradiation with or without ADT • Electroporation with or without ADT
	Cancer has spread to another area of the body (metastasized)	• Advanced treatment required

After prostate surgery

If you have PSA persistence or PSA recurrence and your initial therapy was radical prostatectomy, your next treatment depends on your surgical test results.

No other cancer found

If your PSA level is up but tests don't find cancer in lymph nodes in the pelvis or anywhere else in the body, the preferred treatment is radiation therapy (EBRT) with or without hormone therapy. Monitoring is an option for certain individuals.

Cancer found in lymph nodes

If tests find cancer in lymph nodes in the pelvis, then you may be given radiation therapy, possibly combined with hormone therapy. Additional therapy with another hormone drug may also be included.

Cancer found in another area of the body

If tests find that cancer has spread to another area of the body, it means the cancer has metastasized and needs more advanced treatment. See *NCCN Guidelines for Patients: Advanced-Stage Prostate* Cancer, available at NCCN.org/patientguidelines and on the NCCN Patient Guides for Cancer app.

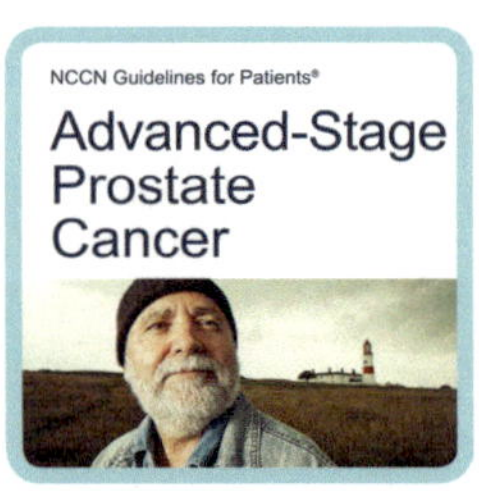

After radiation therapy

If you have PSA recurrence and your initial treatment was radiation therapy, your next treatment depends on your latest test results.

No other cancer found

If your PSA level is up but tests don't find cancer in pelvic lymph nodes or anywhere else in the body, you should undergo another biopsy or simply be monitored with regular testing.

Cancer in the prostate (with or without cancer in pelvic lymph nodes)

If tests find cancer in the prostate and your initial treatment was radiation therapy, monitoring might be an option if the risks seem low. Active treatment typically involves androgen deprivation therapy (ADT) or local therapy, or both.

If cancer is also found in lymph nodes in the pelvis, another hormone drug can be added to ADT or local therapy. If necessary, a radical prostatectomy with removal of the pelvic lymph nodes may be done.

Local therapies

Local therapies focus energy on cancer cells or small tumors while avoiding nearby healthy organs or tissue.

Local therapies are designed to be less aggressive than treatments like surgery or radiation therapy. And they might be less likely to cause side effects like erectile dysfunction or urinary incontinence.

But because the energy from local therapies doesn't travel far or wide, they're only used in certain cases of prostate cancer, particularly in people whose estimated life expectancy is more than 5 years.

Local therapy may be given together with hormone therapy for a more complete result.

Local therapies for persistent or recurrent prostate cancer include:

- **Cryotherapy** – Also known as cryosurgery or cryoablation, cryotherapy destroys cancer cells by freezing them.
- **High-intensity focused ultrasound** – Called HIFU for short, this treatment destroys prostate tissue with heat generated by high-energy ultrasound waves.
- **Re-irradiation** – More radiation—using external beam radiation therapy or internal radiation therapy (brachytherapy)—aims to reach all the cancer in the prostate.
- **Electroporation** – This treatment transmits quick zaps of high-voltage electricity to destroy tumor cells.

Cancer found in another area of the body

If tests find that cancer has spread to another area of the body, that means the cancer has metastasized and needs more advanced treatment. See *NCCN Guidelines for Patients: Advanced-Stage Prostate Cancer*.

Survivorship

Survivorship focuses on the health and well-being of a person with cancer, from diagnosis until the end of life. This includes the physical, mental, emotional, social, and financial effects that begin at diagnosis, continue through treatment, and arise afterward.

Survivorship also includes concerns about follow-up care, late effects of treatment, cancer recurrence, and quality of life. Support from family members, friends, and caregivers is also an important part of survivorship.

Read more about survivorship in *NCCN Guidelines for Patients: Survivorship Care for Healthy Living* and *Survivorship Care for Cancer-Related Late and Long-Term Effects*, available at NCCN.org/patientguidelines and on the NCCN Patient Guides for Cancer app.

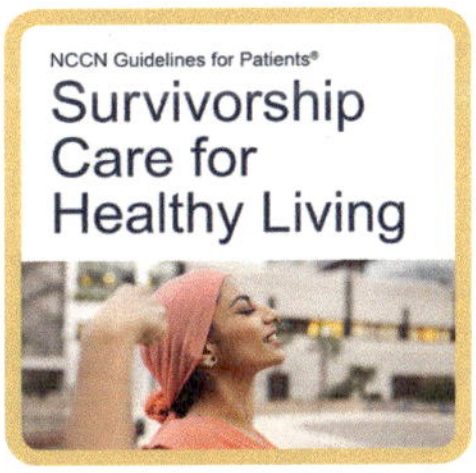

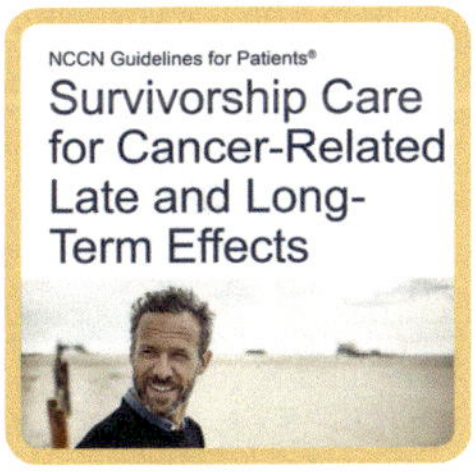

Key points

- After treatment for prostate cancer, some people have prostate-specific antigen (PSA) persistence (the level doesn't drop low enough) or PSA recurrence (the level drops buts starts to rise again).
- PSA persistence and PSA recurrence may be signs that cancer hasn't fully gone away or that it may come back in other parts of the body.
- If you have PSA persistence or recurrence and a life expectancy of 5 years or less, observation may be a more reasonable option than undergoing treatment.
- If tests find that cancer has spread to another area of the body, that means the cancer has metastasized and needs more advanced treatment.
- You can have prostate cancer and still enjoy life after diagnosis and treatment.

Questions to ask

- Why do you believe that my cancer has come back?
- Should I also see a medical oncologist or a radiation oncologist, depending on the next treatment I have?
- If radiation therapy didn't stop the cancer the first time, why should I have it again?
- What are the benefits and risks of adding hormone therapy to radiation therapy?

Survivorship begins at diagnosis. It focuses on your health and well-being before, during, and after your treatment.

Support from family members, friends, and caregivers is an important part of survivorship.

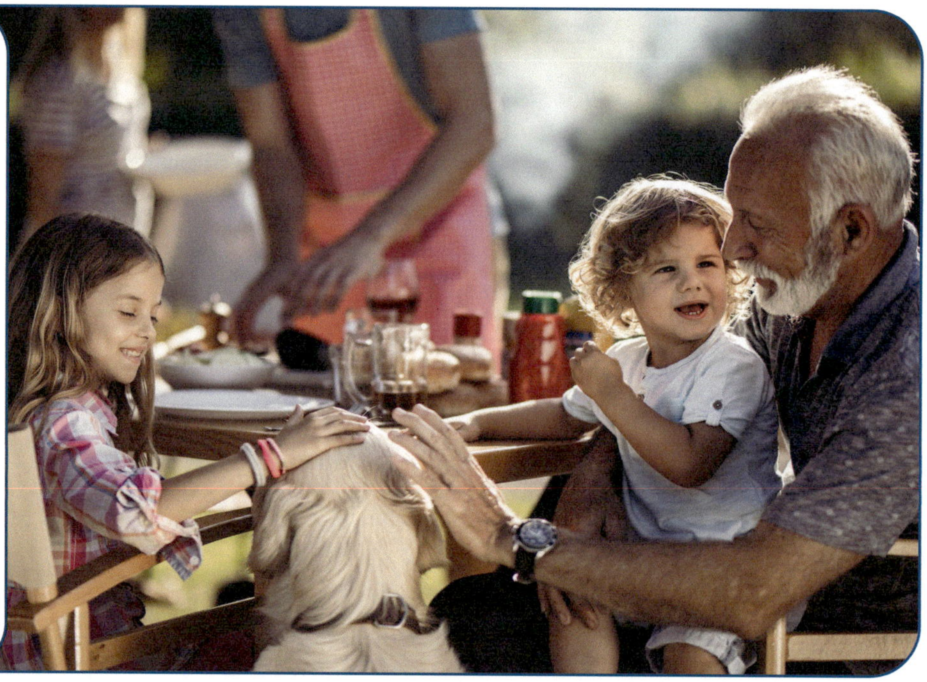

What's next?

After you've been treated for PSA persistence or PSA recurrence, you'll continue to have tests and visits to treat your existing cancer or to watch out for cancer to return.

Surveillance is a key part of your follow-up plan. Be sure to continue to go to follow-up visits and stay in touch with your treatment team.

If the cancer comes back again but doesn't spread beyond the pelvis, you can continue to have treatment for PSA persistence/recurrence.

If the cancer comes back again but has spread to another area of the body, you'll need more advanced treatment. See *NCCN Guidelines for Patients: Advanced-Stage Prostate Cancer*. As always, you can ask about joining a clinical trial.

It's common to feel frustration, anger, regret, despair, and uncertainty—even all at the same time. Know that you can have prostate cancer and still enjoy living after diagnosis and treatment.

Try to take as much pleasure in life as possible. Talk with family or friends. Join a support group to learn how other people are dealing with their cancer. Or talk to your doctor or another member of your care team. They can point you to professionals who can help you deal with these feelings and guide you toward your next steps.

8

Other resources

Want to learn more? Here's how you can get additional help.

What else to know

This guide helps you know your options so you can make informed decisions and improve your cancer care. But it's not the only resource that you have.

Ask for as much information and help as you need. Many people are interested in learning more about:

- Help with choosing the right treatment
- Risks of urinary incontinence and sexual side effects
- Getting a second opinion on your test results or treatment plan
- Dealing with fears, anxiety, or hopelessness
- Talking with others who have prostate cancer

What else to do

Your health care center can help you with next steps. It often has on-site resources to help meet your needs and find answers to your questions. Health care centers can also inform you of resources in your community.

In addition to help from your providers, the resources listed in the next section provide support for many people like yourself.

Where to get help

Look through the list below and visit the provided websites to learn more about these organizations.

AnCan Foundation
ancan.org

Bag It
bagitcancer.org

Cancare, Inc.
cancare.org

Cancer*Care*
cancercare.org

Cancer Hope Network
cancerhopenetwork.org

Cancer Survivor Care
cancersurvivorcare.org

FORCE: Facing Our Risk of Cancer Empowered
facingourrisk.org

GRACE
cancergrace.org

Imerman Angels
imermanangels.org

Malecare
malecare.org

My Faulty Gene
myfaultygene.org

National Alliance of State Prostate Cancer Coalitions (NASPCC)
naspcc.org

PAN Foundation
panfoundation.org

Prostate Conditions Education Council (PCEC)
prostateconditions.org

Prostate Health Education Network (PHEN)
prostatehealthed.org

Triage Cancer
triagecancer.org

ZERO Prostate Cancer
zerocancer.org

Questions to ask

- Are you suggesting options other than what NCCN recommends? If yes, why?
- Will I need PSA tests, digital rectal exams, and biopsies for the rest of my life?
- What will happen if I do nothing?
- If I have an inherited risk for prostate cancer, does that mean my children are going to have cancer, too?
- How do I get a second opinion?

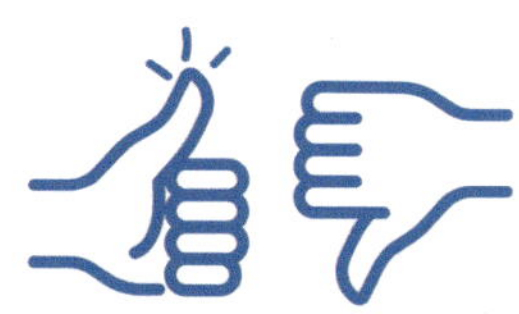

Let us know what you think!

Please take a moment to complete an online survey about the NCCN Guidelines for Patients.
NCCN.org/patients/response

Words to know

active surveillance
Frequent and ongoing testing to watch for changes in cancer status so treatment can be started if needed.

androgen deprivation therapy (ADT)
Hormone therapy that stops the body from making testosterone or blocks cancer cells from using testosterone. ADT can be given through drugs or surgery.

anti-androgen
A drug that stops the action of the hormone testosterone.

biomarker
A biomarker is something found in your body that can be measured to provide information about your health.

biopsy
A procedure that removes fluid or tissue samples to be tested for disease.

brachytherapy
A treatment with radiation from an object placed near or in the tumor. Also called internal radiation.

castration
Surgery that removes the testicles, or drugs that suppress the function of the testicles, to minimize testosterone levels.

computed tomography (CT)
An imaging test that uses x-rays from many angles to make cross-sectional images of the inside of the body.

digital rectal exam
An exam of the prostate by feeling it through the wall of the rectum.

early-stage prostate cancer
Prostate cancer that usually grows slowly and stays within the prostate.

enlarged prostate
An overgrowth of tissue in the prostate that isn't caused by cancer. Also sometimes called benign prostatic hyperplasia.

erectile dysfunction
A lack of blood flow to the penis that limits getting or staying erect.

external beam radiation therapy (EBRT)
A treatment in which a machine outside the body aims radiation precisely at cancer inside the body.

germline mutation
A genetic change that is passed from a parent to their biological child(ren). Also called an inheredited mutation.

Gleason score
A rating of how much prostate cancer cells look like normal cells under the microscope.

Grade Group
Like a Gleason score, a Grade Group is a rating of how much prostate cancer cells look like normal cells under the microscope. Grade Groups are meant to be easier to use than Gleason scores.

hormone therapy
A cancer treatment that stops the making or action of hormones. Also called androgen deprivation therapy.

life expectancy
An estimate of years a person is likely to live based on statistics of other people in similar circumstances.

luteinizing hormone-releasing hormone (LHRH) agonist
A drug that stops the testicles from making testosterone.

luteinizing hormone-releasing hormone (LHRH) antagonist
A drug that acts in the brain to stop the testicles from making testosterone.

lymph nodes
Small, bean-shaped structures that contain disease-fighting cells. Hundreds of lymph nodes are located throughout the body.

magnetic resonance imaging (MRI)
An imaging test that uses radio waves and powerful magnets to make pictures of the insides of the body.

metastasis
The spread of cancer from the site where it started to a new site in the body.

nomogram
A mathematical tool that uses health information to predict an outcome.

observation
A period of watching for cancer growth or occurrence while not receiving treatment.

orchiectomy
An operation to reduce testosterone in the body by removing one or both testicles.

palliative care
Health care for the symptoms of cancer and the side effects of cancer treatment. Also called supportive care.

pathologist
A doctor who specializes in testing cells and tissue to find disease.

pelvic lymph node dissection
An operation that removes lymph nodes in the pelvis.

perineum
The body region between the scrotum and anus.

positron emission tomography (PET)
An imaging test that uses radioactive material to see the shape and function of body parts.

prostate-specific antigen (PSA)
A protein made by the prostate that helps semen transport sperm. PSA is measured in nanograms per milliliter of blood (ng/mL).

PSA density
The level of PSA—a prostate-made protein—in relation to the size of the prostate.

PSA persistence
When PSA level is still detectable after prostate cancer treatment.

PSA recurrence
When PSA level drops after prostate cancer treatment but then rises again.

radiation therapy
Treatment that uses high-energy rays (radiation) to kill cancer cells and stop new cancer cells from being made.

radical prostatectomy
An operation that removes the entire prostate as well as surrounding tissue, seminal vesicles, and sometimes lymph nodes.

recurrence
The return of cancer after a disease-free period.

risk factor
Something that increases the chance of getting a disease.

seminal vesicles
Two glands that make and store part of the fluid that becomes semen.

somatic mutation
A non-hereditary change in your DNA that occurred after conception. Also called an acquired mutation.

staging
The process of rating the extent of cancer in the body.

supportive care
Health care that supports the physical, emotional, social, and spiritual needs of patients, families, and caregivers. Also called palliative care.

surgical margin
The normal-looking tissue around a tumor that is removed during an operation.

testosterone
The main hormone that controls male sexual development and physical characteristics.

urethra
A tube that carries urine from the bladder to outside of the body through the penis. It also expels semen.

urinary incontinence
A condition in which the release of urine can't be controlled.

We want your feedback!

Our goal is to provide helpful and easy-to-understand information on cancer. Take our survey to let us know what we got right and what we could do better.
NCCN.org/patients/feedback

NCCN Contributors

This patient guide is based on the NCCN Clinical Practice Guidelines in Oncology (NCCN Guidelines®) for Prostate Cancer, Version 5.2026. It was adapted, reviewed, and published with help from the following people:

Dorothy A. Shead, MS
Senior Director
Patient Information Operations

John Murphy
Senior Medical Writer

Lisa Diehl
Production Layout Artist

The NCCN Clinical Practice Guidelines in Oncology (NCCN Guidelines®) for Prostate Cancer, Version 5.2026 were developed by the following NCCN Panel Members:

Daniel E. Spratt, MD/Chair
Case Comprehensive Cancer Center/ University Hospitals Seidman Cancer Center and Cleveland Clinic Taussig Cancer Institute

Sandy Srinivas, MD/Vice-Chair
Stanford Cancer Institute

Nabil Adra, MD, MSc
Indiana University Melvin and Bren Simon Comprehensive Cancer Center

Bilawal Ahmed, MD
The University of Tennessee Health Science Center

Yi An, MD
Yale Cancer Center/Smilow Cancer Hospital

Rhonda Bitting, MD
Duke Cancer Institute

Brian Chapin, MD
The University of Texas MD Anderson Cancer Center

Heather H. Cheng, MD, PhD
Fred Hutchinson Cancer Center

Steve Y. Cho, MD
University of Wisconsin Carbone Cancer Center

Anthony Victor D'Amico, MD, PhD
Dana-Farber/Brigham and Women's Cancer Center | Mass General Cancer Center

Neil Desai, MD, MHS
UT Southwestern Simmons Comprehensive Cancer Center

Tanya Dorff, MD
City of Hope National Cancer Center

James A. Eastham, MD
Memorial Sloan Kettering Cancer Center Institute

Thomas A. Farrington, BSEE
Prostate Health Education Network (PHEN)

Xin Gao, MD
Dana-Farber/Brigham and Women's Cancer Center | Mass General Cancer Center

Shilpa Gupta, MD
Case Comprehensive Cancer Center/ University Hospitals Seidman Cancer Center and Cleveland Clinic Taussig Cancer Institute

Joseph E. Ippolito, MD, PhD
Siteman Cancer Center at Barnes-Jewish Hospital and Washington University School of Medicine

R. Jeffrey Karnes, MD
Mayo Clinic Comprehensive Cancer Center

Amar Kishan, MD
UCLA Jonsson Comprehensive Cancer Center

Michael R. Kuettel, MD, PhD, MBA
Roswell Park Comprehensive Cancer Center

Joshua M. Lang, MD, MS
University of Wisconsin Carbone Cancer Center

*Daniel Lee, MD, MS
Abramson Cancer Center at The University of Pennsylvania

Tamara Lotan, MD
Johns Hopkins Kimmel Cancer Center

*Andrew McDonald, MD, MS
O'Neal Comprehensive Cancer Center at UAB

Todd Morgan, MD
University of Michigan Rogel Cancer Center

Rodrigo Pessoa, MD, PhD
Moffitt Cancer Center

Soroush Rais-Bahrami, MD, MBA
O'Neal Comprehensive Cancer Center at UAB

Mack Roach, III, MD
UCSF Helen Diller Family Comprehensive Cancer Center

Tyler Robin, MD, PhD
University of Colorado Cancer Center

*Stan Rosenfeld
University of California San Francisco Patient Services Committee Chair

*Kristen R. Scarpato, MD, MPH
Vanderbilt-Ingram Cancer Center

*Tyler Seibert, MD, PhD
UC San Diego Moores Cancer Center

*Ahmad Shabsigh, MD
The Ohio State University Comprehensive Cancer Center - James Cancer Hospital and Solove Research Institute

Russell Szmulewitz, MD
The UChicago Medicine Comprehensive Cancer Center

Benjamin A. Teply, MD
Fred & Pamela Buffett Cancer Center

Jonathan Tward, MD, PhD
Huntsman Cancer Institute at the University of Utah

Richard Valicenti, MD
UC Davis Comprehensive Cancer Center

David VanderWeele, MD, PhD
Robert H. Lurie Comprehensive Cancer Center of Northwestern University

Jessica Karen Wong, MD
Fox Chase Cancer Center

NCCN

Deborah Freedman-Cass, PhD
Senior Manager
Clinical Content Operations

Emily Kovach
Guidelines Layout Specialist

* Reviewed this patient guide. For disclosures, visit NCCN.org/disclosures.

NCCN Cancer Centers

For contact information, visit NCCN.org/cancercenters.

Abramson Cancer Center
at the University of Pennsylvania
Philadelphia, Pennsylvania

Case Comprehensive Cancer Center/
University Hospitals Seidman Cancer Center and
Cleveland Clinic Taussig Cancer Institute
Cleveland, Ohio

City of Hope National Medical Center
Duarte, California

Dana-Farber/Brigham and Women's Cancer Center |
Mass General Cancer Center
Boston, Massachusetts

Duke Cancer Institute
Durham, North Carolina

Fox Chase Cancer Center
Philadelphia, Pennsylvania

Fred & Pamela Buffett Cancer Center
Omaha, Nebraska

Fred Hutchinson Cancer Center
Seattle, Washington

Huntsman Cancer Institute at the University of Utah
Salt Lake City, Utah

Indiana University Melvin and Bren Simon
Comprehensive Cancer Center
Indianapolis, Indiana

Johns Hopkins Kimmel Cancer Center
Baltimore, Maryland

Mayo Clinic Comprehensive Cancer Center
Phoenix/Scottsdale, Arizona
Jacksonville, Florida
Rochester, Minnesota

Memorial Sloan Kettering Cancer Center
New York, New York

Moffitt Cancer Center
Tampa, Florida

O'Neal Comprehensive Cancer Center at UAB
Birmingham, Alabama

Robert H. Lurie Comprehensive Cancer Center
of Northwestern University
Chicago, Illinois

Roswell Park Comprehensive Cancer Center
Buffalo, New York

Siteman Cancer Center at Barnes-Jewish Hospital
and Washington University School of Medicine
St. Louis, Missouri

St. Jude Children's Research Hospital/
The University of Tennessee Health Science Center
Memphis, Tennessee

Stanford Cancer Institute
Stanford, California

The Ohio State University Comprehensive Cancer Center -
James Cancer Hospital and Solove Research Institute
Columbus, Ohio

The UChicago Medicine Comprehensive Cancer Center
Chicago, Illinois

The University of Texas MD Anderson Cancer Center
Houston, Texas

UC Davis Comprehensive Cancer Center
Sacramento, California

UC San Diego Moores Cancer Center
La Jolla, California

UCLA Jonsson Comprehensive Cancer Center
Los Angeles, California

UCSF Helen Diller Family Comprehensive Cancer Center
San Francisco, California

University of Colorado Cancer Center
Aurora, Colorado

University of Michigan Rogel Cancer Center
Ann Arbor, Michigan

University of Wisconsin Carbone Cancer Center
Madison, Wisconsin

UT Southwestern Simmons
Comprehensive Cancer Center
Dallas, Texas

Vanderbilt-Ingram Cancer Center
Nashville, Tennessee

Yale Cancer Center/Smilow Cancer Hospital
New Haven, Connecticut

Notes

Index

share with us.

Take our survey and help make the NCCN Guidelines for Patients better for everyone!

NCCN.org/patients/comments

Made in United States
Cleveland, OH
25 April 2026

36196917R00050